Licensed to Prac

The role of the staff n

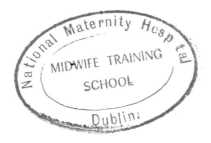

Licensed to Practise

The role of the staff nurse

Mary Sykes BA, SRN, SCM, RNT

Director of Nursing Services at
St James's University Hospital, Leeds

Her team of contributors is drawn from
Leeds Eastern District Health Authority

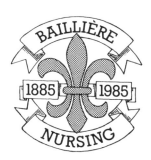

Baillière Tindall London Philadelphia Toronto
Mexico City Rio de Janeiro Sydney Tokyo Hong Kong

Baillière Tindall   1 St Anne's Road
W. B. Saunders   Eastbourne, East Sussex BN21 3UN,
                     England

                     West Washington Square
                     Philadelphia, PA 19105, USA

                     1 Goldthorne Avenue
                     Toronto, Ontario M8Z 5T9, Canada

                     Apartado 26370—Cedro 512
                     Mexico 4, DF Mexico

                     Rua Evaristo da Veiga, 55, 20° andar
                     Rio de Janeiro—RJ, Brazil

                     ABP Australia Ltd,
                     44–50 Waterloo Road
                     North Ryde, NSW 2113, Australia

                     Ichibancho Central Building,
                     22-1 Ichibancho
                     Chiyoda-ku, Tokyo 102, Japan

                     10/fl, Inter-Continental Plaza,
                     94 Granville Road
                     Tsim Sha Tsui East, Kowloon,
                     Hong Kong

First published 1985

Typeset by Scribe Design, Gillingham, Kent
Printed in Great Britain by Billing & Sons Ltd, Worcester

British Library Cataloguing in Publication Data

Licensed to practise: the role of the staff nurse.
  1. Nursing—Great Britain
  I. Sykes, Mary
  610.73'06'92   RT11

  ISBN 0–7020–1087–1

Contents

Foreword

In recent years increasing attention has been directed towards the role and performance expectations of the newly qualified nurse—the Staff Nurse. Basic nurse education aims to produce a registered nurse who demonstrates a range of competencies determined by a field of practice and syllabus of training. However, such a statement begs one to question the meaning of competence. The time was that a nurse on qualifying was expected to be capable of performing the full range of activities of a trained nurse with little or no consideration being given to the newness of the role. There were, and probably are, some newly qualified nurses who, in the flush of excitement and glory, felt they could perform the full range of activities *until* faced with the reality of the expectations of this new role.

What are those expectations? To whom do the expectations relate—self, peers, students, patients, relatives? Each has expectations of a Staff Nurse which differ from those held for a senior student nurse. What are appropriate role expectations of a newly qualified nurse? Is it realistic to expect such a nurse to fulfil the full range of Staff Nurse responsibilities to the same level of competence as the experienced Staff Nurse? An interesting qualitative component has been introduced. Previously the discussion centred on demonstrating a range of competencies, now it is suggested that there may be a difference in the *level* of competency between the newly qualified and the experienced Staff Nurse.

It is the transition in the level of competency that this book addresses. In identifying the differing role requirements and expectations of the Staff Nurse, the contributors highlight the varied facets of the role and the problems and difficulties which might be encountered by the new Staff Nurse. As indicated earlier, increasing attention is being directed towards this transition phase. Following the establishment of experimental Staff Nurse development programmes in 1982, the evaluation of which is still awaited, many health authorities have taken their own initiatives. Staff Nurse development, and in particular constructive help and guidance in steering the new Staff Nurse through the transition to the confident and competent experienced Staff Nurse, is now considered a priority issue in many Continuing Education and In-Service Training Departments.

The issues raised in this book and the advice and guidance offered by contributors experienced in working with newly qualified nurses should prove a considerable asset to those embarking on their first appointment as Registered Nurses. Furthermore the book gives valuable reminders and insights to experienced clinical nurses and teachers of the apprehensions, problems and difficulties experienced or perceived by the new Staff Nurse. For this reason I would recommend the book to all qualifying nurses, whether they be newly registered or working with the newly registered. The wealth of case material well demonstrates the goals that have yet to be achieved.

J.D. Duberley
MSc, SRN, RSCN, RCNT
Regional Nurse
Professional Practice
Education and Development

Preface

A magic formula for success is not handed out with Registration—it has to be worked at. We have attempted to define some of the basic principles which hold true even in this period of rapid change, and to set thoughts on pathways for further development and reading.

Relationships and maintaining safe patient care are priorities, but hopefully the ensuing chapters will help the reader to grasp something of the enormously complex, all-embracing art that is good nursing care.

Each contributor has a different style, chapters 1, 2, 3 and 4 being discursive as befits their subjects, the rest having a more direct and academic presentation for more factual matters. We hope these changes in tempo enhance rather than detract from your enjoyment and benefit.

There is a little overlap, but it is felt important to preserve each chapter to be read in isolation if required.

Mary Sykes

Contributors

Jenny Dale trained at St James's Hospital, Leeds and became a Staff Nurse in an acute medical ward followed by a year on a cardiothoracic surgical ward. Jenny then went to work in a large general hospital in Ottawa, Canada. On returning home she trained in midwifery at St James's University Hospital and is now a Staff Midwife there.

Lawrence Whyte began RMN training in 1973 at St Augustine's Hospital, Kent. He then completed a post registration SRN course at Kent and Canterbury Hospital before returning to psychiatric nursing. From 1979 to 1982 he left nursing to complete a BA (Hons) Sociology at the University of Kent. At present he is working as a Charge Nurse in Acute Psychiatry at St James's University Hospital, Leeds whilst studying part time for an MA in Health Service Studies at the Nuffield Centre, University of Leeds. He has written several articles for nursing journals specializing in the topics of health service policy and issues within the nursing of the mentally ill.

June Gingell qualified from Luton and Dunstable Hospital as a State Registered Nurse in 1972 and worked as a Staff Nurse on wards specializing in chest diseases. June qualified as a midwife in 1975 at St James's University Hospital, working as a qualified midwife for a period of 8 months. A post as Sister on a medical ward followed—the ward was a pilot ward for implementing the Nursing Process and in 1980 a form of primary nursing was instituted. In 1980 June made a study trip to Colorado, the aim being to examine how the Nursing Process and primary nursing was implemented there. She has had articles on both these subjects published and since 1981 has worked as Nursing Process Co-ordinator at St James's University Hospital, working closely with the Ward Sisters and the Department of Continuing Education.

Mia Telford has held a variety of posts ranging from theatre work to health visiting and infection control nursing. Having always been interested in law she studied for a BA whilst at home caring for young children and is currently a student on the Law Society Final Course with a view to becoming a solicitor. At the time of writing she was Control of Infection Nursing Officer at St James's University Hospital, Leeds.

Christine Matthewson after completing an honours degree in French at Durham University, worked briefly as an auxiliary in a small hospital in Hackney before training at St Thomas's Hospital, London. She remained there as a Staff Nurse for several years before going to Exeter to study midwifery. After further staffing experience in Exeter, Carlisle and Leeds she took up her present post of Second Sister on a professorial medical ward, St James's University Hospital, Leeds in April 1983.

Susan Cottam started nursing in the early 1960s, and after breaking off to have a family, returned eight years later. Her main area of work since qualifying has been medicine. Her current post is that of Sister-in-charge of a professorial medical ward at St James's University Hospital, Leeds. For the past year she has been the chairwoman of the Nursing Process Working Party for St James's and other hospitals in the District.

Vivien Coates graduated and became a State Registered Nurse from Newcastle Polytechnic in 1980. She then undertook a two year research project on nutrition of hospital patients at St James's University Hospital, Leeds, funded by the Yorkshire Regional Health Authority. She was awarded an MPhil for this work. Since then she has worked as a Staff Nurse on general medical and plastic surgery wards, and is currently working on a general surgical ward. The research project is about to be published by the Royal College of Nursing in their Research Series, and she has also written several other articles.

Simon Old trained at Leeds Polytechnic in conjunction with St James's University Hospital, Leeds and was awarded a BSc

Nursing Degree with commendation in 1980. He was appointed as Research Nurse to a DHSS funded project in 1982, having previously gained clinical experience as a Staff Nurse. The project is concerned with evaluation of computerized monitoring in the intensive care environment. Through his work, he has developed a keen interest in the use of computers in nursing. He does not claim to be a computer specialist but firmly believes that computer technology has a lot to offer nurses and nursing.

Angela Senior trained in Edinburgh, where she worked as a Staff Nurse prior to moving to London for midwifery training. She has travelled widely throughout her native Caribbean and Africa and has worked in the field of nurse education in both Ghana and Kenya before coming to St James's University Hospital, Leeds in 1974. She has since held posts of Clinical Teacher, Nurse Tutor and presently Senior Tutor Continuing Education. She is committed to developing and maintaining the professional status of the nurse and sees continuing education as the major key.

Mary Sykes has had a variety of posts including midwife, sister of a surgical ward, teacher and nurse manager. She has had several articles published and edited *Gastroenterology for Nurses* in 1982 for Pitman Medical Press. She is Director of Acute Nursing at St James's University Hospital, Leeds.

Thoughts of a Newly Qualified Staff Nurse

Jennifer Dale

So here I am, a Staff Nurse. I sat and read the results of my examinations three times before it finally sank in and then the feeling of pride that swept over me was immense. 'Staff Nurse Dale'. Oh, how I had climbed the social ladder that day!

My parents and friends were overjoyed of course but I wondered if anyone from outside the hospital environment had any insight into the role of the Staff Nurse. Come to think of it, did I? I had a couple of days off so I went on a shopping spree I could ill afford and bought a new silver buckle and white shoes. The expense did not matter; after all, one could not be a 'proper' Staff Nurse without all of the trimmings could one?

During those days before returning to duty I also tried to think about this new rank in life that I had achieved. I felt a little overawed but also looked forward to the long-hoped-for glamour of being a qualified nurse. Everything was going to be so different now; after all Staff Nurses are important aren't they?

My big day arrived. My first day as a Staff Nurse. I floated on to the ward in my brand new uniform trying to look dignified as I felt this befitted the title – I might add aided by an extra hour in front of the mirror working on my appearance. Everyone made a fuss over my uniform and I preened in front of them like any fashion model, but the rest of the day was to prove less glamorous and my dignity far from intact.

Chapter 1

I took the report on the patients from the morning staff and here my worries began. Every minor problem the patients had that I might have to make a decision about became major setbacks to me. Constipated? Urinary tract infection? I had dealt with these problems many times but now seemed to lack confidence in my own judgement. The patients of course put great faith in me due to the uniform I was wearing. Couldn't they see it was brand new, straight from the sewing room, with *me* in it? Their endless questions frightened me. How much of what I knew should I tell them? Was it my duty to do so? I fumbled my way through my answers, always fearful I might say the wrong thing. When the relatives came along to ask about their loved ones I wanted to make a quick exit to the staff room to avoid further questions. As a student it is so easy to pass awkward questions along to the nurse in charge, but that was me! Oh to have my student uniform to hide in for the rest of the day.

I hovered over the student nurses like an old hen feeling I had to watch everthing they were doing. I knew this was silly and something I had always hated myself but I could not help it. The other problem of course was the students themselves. How should I treat them? I had always said as a student nurse that when I qualified I would not become 'one of them', but here I was feeling totally alien to them. Half of me wanted to be accepted as one of the girls but the other half wanted to see that glimmer of respect a Staff Nurse receives. I knew of course that one does not obtain respect with the donning of a white uniform but when did this change begin?

My idea of being a good Staff Nurse that morning was to allocate the patients, organize coffee breaks, keep the nursing station immaculate, and await the doctors. Oh dear, what a disaster! My first ward round with the doctors: I spent hours memorizing all the latest results and putting all the X-rays in order in the trolley. In fact I was so absorbed in the latter that the doctors set off on their own without me! I was humiliated. But when I caught up with them I was further embarrassed by my inability to answer a question about a patient's sputum. Sputum! No blood results, no X-rays, just plain old sputum and I couldn't answer. Where had I gone wrong?

I handed over the report to the night staff and then could not get off to sleep that night for fear I had left something out. For Staff Nurses do not miss anything, do they?

There were so many such problems during the months ahead and I always wished there was a guideline to help me through. Not as a replacement to experience, which of course there will never be, but to make me feel I was not alone in this feeling of inadequacy. I came to the conclusion that my treasured white uniform labelled me as someone responsible and wished my silver buckle could be replaced by 'L' plates during my first fumbling weeks. I cannot remember the time when I began performing the daily role of Staff Nurse or announced myself on the 'phone without mumbling but I do know it was not the day I passed my exams...

Student Nurse–Staff Nurse: What is the Difference?

Christine Matthewson

National Maternity Hospital
MIDWIFE TRAINING
SCHOOL
Dublin.

You are a third-year student – a valuable member of the ward team who no doubt receives a modicum of respect from the 'lower ranks' for your superior knowledge and experience. You probably know all the Staff Nurses pretty well by now and you may feel you've related well to Sister – she trusts you and you respect her. You're doing fine. You have taken your finals. You've passed. What is so different about you? As you set foot on your new ward in full regalia, determined to be the best Staff Nurse in the hospital, what magical metamorphosis has occurred? The answer is simple. Nothing is different. Nothing has changed. For the time being *you* are obviously exactly the same. The difference is in how other people see you and what they expect of you. In time as you adapt to these expectations you will develop new skills – perhaps a slightly different attitude. Change is inevitable. But it does not come overnight.

Think back to your first ward. Can you remember when you got rid of that horrible lost feeling? Or even your second ward. You expected to settle down there more quickly but it was still awful at first – everything was so different and in some ways you felt just as lost all over again. In fact, when you think about it, you always feel lost when you start a new allocation and that doesn't change just because you are a Staff Nurse. You can't take a temperature until you know where the thermometers are kept any more than you can set up for insertion of a CVP line until you find the CSSD room.

There is no single model for 'super staff' but there are a few points to remember which might help:

1 You are qualified – therefore competent. Enjoy it. Relax. You will teach by example almost without knowing it.
2 Be adaptable. You will have to work in many different areas – take what you can from each. In any given area you will have many tasks to perform – some complex and obviously related to your training. Other more menial tasks may be equally important: mopping the floor in the interests of ward safety, making tea as a gesture of comfort.
3 Be open and approachable. You no longer have your own six to ten patients to care for in isolation. You have the whole ward, their friends and relatives as well as all your learners and auxiliaries, your fellow Staff Nurses, medical and paramedical staff, domestic staff – in fact anyone who sets foot on the ward lays claim to your attention. It is your task now, as a Staff Nurse, to draw all the threads together in order to provide the best possible care for your patients and the best possible working and learning environment for your learners. The key to success lies in the art of communication which involves listening just as much as talking.

Let us return to consider the changes that will inevitably take place now that you have qualified. Those you are caring for and working with see you differently and it is in your relations with them that you will develop the skills which mark you out as a capable Staff Nurse. Most senior students seem to worry about the same things when contemplating their change in role. Generally they feel competent to administer patient care. Although apprehensive they feel they are able to handle a crisis. What worries them is the thought of dealing with difficult questions from patients or relatives and the problem of paperwork, which form to fill in when, the difficulty of obtaining obscure items urgently needed at short notice. They are also concerned about telling people what to do without seeming 'bossy' and trusting others to administer care as competently as they would themselves without 'nagging' or 'snooping'. I will now consider 'the Staff Nurse' as seen through the eyes of the various people with whom she is in contact in an attempt to pinpoint some of the problem areas, and to offer some practical advice where possible.

Patients

You are qualified – therefore you immediately inspire confidence. If you are giving practical care your patient knows he will be left comfortable; his every need will be met; everything will be done to ensure his safety and well-being. This is a daunting thought yet you rightfully gain satisfaction and confidence from your expertise. Having such faith in your practical skills the patient expects much more of you than of a student. As an experienced nurse you understand why he is feeling ill and what is causing his pain. You must have nursed others with his condition. Can you explain his disease to him simply and lucidly? Which investigations will be done? Will they be lengthy and painful? What treatment is possible? How long might he be in hospital? He is far more likely to ask you all these questions rather than the dreaded 'Have I got cancer, nurse?'

If a patient fears he has cancer the apprehension can be seen building up over a period of days. The doctors may have talked to him and as far as they are concerned they have told him he has a terminal disease, but often patients fail to understand, either because the language goes over their heads or because they really don't want to know. In my experience, if they ask outright, they want to know the truth. If possible you can give them the opportunity to ask when they have a close relative with them so they are not left alone with their thoughts afterwards. However, some people are so protective of close family they prefer to face the consequences alone. Alternatively, some families will do everything possible to keep the diagnosis from the patient. This can lead to a lot of strain with everyone secretly knowing the truth, yet still pretending things are fine. As nurses, we can only give advice and the benefit of experience – we must still be guided by the wishes of the patient or his family.

Because you have considerable knowledge and are able to explain his illness to him the patient will confide in you and you must develop your professional integrity, learning to distinguish between the things you must pass on to nursing or medical colleagues and the things you must hold in confidence between the patient and yourself. There is a great need for impartiality. Whatever your patient confides to you, you are not his judge. Your skills are in healing mind as well as body but you are not a morally superior being. You are simply using your health and strength to fill his shortfall. The confidence your patients show in you does in time give you confidence in yourself. I am sure patients, so full of gratitude for what we do for them, never begin to realize what they do for us!

In order to understand your patient's position fully you may have to come to terms with a culture completely alien to your own. You must do your best (using his family or hospital interpreters for communication) to ensure he and his family know what is happening. For example, if he has an infectious disease everyone must understand the reasons for wearing gowns or masks and washing hands after visiting. There may be dietary laws or special religious observances he has to make, however ill he is. You must be aware of their importance to his general well-being. It's no good saying 'he won't eat hospital food'. Can his relatives not bring food in? Do they know it must be salt or sugar free?

The dilemma for the Staff Nurse is that while each individual expects more of her she finds she has total responsibility for more patients than ever before, yet has less time to give to each one. She is continually called away to answer the telephone, to speak to relatives, to talk to the other health care professionals; everybody wants the nurse in charge. She may no longer have the luxury of an uninterrupted half hour with her patient, gradually building up a rapport with him as she washes and shaves him. She has to form contact much more quickly but without superficiality. She will undoubtedly look back longingly on the days when she could close the curtains behind her and be left to her work in peace.

Learners

The whole of chapter 3 will be devoted to the relationship between Staff Nurse and learner. Suffice it to say that the learners look to you as someone with more experience and knowledge than they; someone who will supervise, teach and assess them. They look to you to provide a framework of organization for their days. They expect information from you regarding changes in the treatment or condition of their patients. They also expect solidarity from you, a newly qualified Staff Nurse, so recently 'one of them'; they expect you to have more insight into their problems than the more senior qualified staff. Once you are able to relax a little you become more aware of other people's needs and fears and you will soon know which nurses you can rely on to look after their patients competently and which require closer supervision; which can be depended on both to notice and report a change in their patients' condition and those whose judgement is not yet sufficiently formed. You will learn the unfortunate necessity of asking people to do exactly what you want. Saying 'keep a close eye on him' is meaningless. 'Keep him on bed-rest, take his pulse and blood pressure half-hourly and watch for any signs of bleeding from the puncture site in his left groin' is much less open to misinterpretation. You will find that people *expect* you to direct them, which soon makes you feel less 'bossy'. There are obviously ways of asking or telling people to do things. It is perfectly possible to be authoritative and pleasant at the same time.

Senior nurses

Sister will expect your loyalty and support. I have never had to work for a Sister I did not respect, which has made loyalty easy. These days, when staffing posts are not so easy to come by, one may not always have the choice of where to work. For a happy ward environment, however, it is vital that the trained staff work well together and support one another. As a newly qualified Staff Nurse you are often well placed to liaise between learners and trained staff. This is not 'telling tales'. Sometimes learners are unwilling to bother Sister with their private ailments or concerns but she may be able to help if made aware of their worries; encourage them to confide in her. Sister may insist on a certain procedure being carried out in a practical way – you will be able to explain the reasoning behind the practice.

You are also part of the team which ensures that the ward is well-equipped. It is no longer good enough to moan that 'we haven't any pillows' or 'there are no more giving sets'. You must find out who does the ordering, how often and when. You must notice in advance what is being used so it can be re-ordered in good time. You must find out where things can be obtained urgently without always resorting to simple borrowing, particularly in these days of ward budgeting. There is usually someone available to advise you: your ward clerk, the porters, the liaison officer for stores, even the switchboard. Failing this, a senior nurse will always be to hand, either a covering Nursing Officer or a Staff Nurse from an adjacent ward. Many wards give their trained staff responsibility for stocking a certain store cupboard and in time you become the expert manager in your own area – another boost for the morale.

The Nursing Officer quite simply she expects you to know what's going on. She needs to be told about sickness or staffing problems so she can manage her unit efficiently. She needs to know of any unusual occurence on the ward – accidents and incidents (when in doubt contact her, fill in the appropriate form and make a note in the Kardex). She should be told about critically ill patients who may have relatives wishing to stay overnight. She should also be informed when the local or national celebrities are admitted to your ward so she can notify administration in case they need to deal with the press or the hospital hierarchy. If you are unsure, tell her. Most Nursing Officers these days bend over backwards to help their newly qualified staff. In fact, of the sample of Staff Nurses I spoke to, many particularly mentioned their Nursing Officer as someone who helped them a great deal, who had made a point of being available so that when problems arose and they were in charge and alone they had no qualms about approaching her. If you do face a sudden problem and you need to turn to someone for advice, you are not admitting defeat but simply recognizing your lack of experience and therefore showing your maturity and responsibility.

Doctors

There is no doubt you will have far more dealings with the medical staff once qualified. A simple initial point is to make sure of the hierarchy of doctors on your ward so you are able to contact the right member of the right firm for the right patient. The communication is two-way. You are better placed to know about patients' worries or whether their pain is controlled (they may only see them 'asleep' – you turned the patient three times this morning and know he groaned each time), whether their condition has generally improved or deteriorated overnight, whether they have suddenly spiked a pyrexia or developed a rash. You know about the home situation – whether it is more appropriate for the medical team to talk to husband/wife or son/daughter, whether the patient has elderly relatives or young children to care for on discharge. The doctor obviously has a deeper understanding of the patient's medical condition. Glean what you can from him and pass on what you learn to stimulate the learner's interest. You are also in a better position to answer those 'awkward' questions the patient poses when you have heard the Consultant voicing his thoughts that morning.

A brief word on doctors' rounds. You are there for the benefit of your patient. No matter how many visiting Registrars, medical students, pharmacists, research students and House Officers may be present, your place is right there at your patient's side. This way you can reassure him simply by your presence. After all, he knows you. You will find he often looks at you for support even while he is answering the doctor's questions. You are there to ensure his comfort and privacy. Make sure the curtains are closed when he is examined or questioned. Make sure he is sitting or lying

11

comfortably during the physical examination and that he is left both comfortable and safe when the doctors have finished. Also make sure he knows and understands what they have said to him; you may well have to do a second round once the team has gone in order to ensure this. You are also there to make your observations known. Don't be afraid to speak up. The patient may claim to be eating well at every meal when you know he never touches a morsel. You don't have to contradict him outright. Choose your moment to make sure the medical staff get the right story. You can fill the doctors in on the home situation. A husband with a fit healthy wife will obviously be discharged home more quickly after a myocardial infarction than someone whose wife is wheelchair-bound and dependent on him.

Obviously you are there to gain information too. You want to know what's going to happen next so you can be prepared in advance. Which tests are in the pipeline? When are intravenous infusions and drains to be removed? What have investigations revealed so far? Once you have been on the ward for a while you will be able to predict which nursing observations are needed. The doctors won't say to you 'We want this man on a four-hourly temperature, daily urinalysis for blood and protein, and a stool chart'. They say 'Pyrexial?', 'Anything in the urine?', 'Bowels?' – looking at you enquiringly. You have to know the information they will need before they ask!

If you have a few minutes before a ward round do make sure you have got all the notes and X-rays you will need. The round will run more smoothly. Also have a plan in your mind of which patients are due to be seen just in case the doctors overlook someone. You are then able to retrieve the right patients from the Day Room so they can be near their beds when the doctors arrive. The Houseman is supposed to lead the round but if he is looking lost it will be helpful if you know where to go next.

Once you are qualified, although you are free to read and attend study days, you will find one of the most pleasant ways to learn is to pick the brains of the experts, but don't forget to pass on what you learn, because that makes everyone's task more interesting.

Other health care professionals

You are now dealing with a whole workforce of experts who will be only too pleased when you express interest in their work: physiotherapists, pharmacists, dietitians, occupational therapists, diabetic health visitors, speech therapists, social workers, stoma therapists – any number of people available for you to contact. Again, they expect you to be able to tell them about the patient's physical condition and mental state and something of his social background. They will give you feedback on how the patient is progressing in their area. A ward meeting is an ideal opportunity to discuss the different aspects of progress but it is not always possible to get everyone together. Once more the vital importance of your communication skills is highlighted.

Some of these practitioners will be able to give you more information about the patient's home life so you are more easily able to assess when discharge is feasible. The social worker might be asked to compile a formal social report with details of domestic history, quality of housing, closeness of family ties, etc. This is obviously a confidential document. The occupational therapist and physiotherapist may take the patient on a home visit to see how he performs on his own ground. Between them the occupational therapist, the social worker and social services can arrange for the provision of various home adaptations and fitments or special equipment to help the patient manage in the community. The social worker has a wealth of knowledge and can answer any question your patient may ask about claims for special allowances and so on. She will be able to advise about convalescent homes, day centres, holiday relief schemes and attendance allowances. She will know of the best way of getting full time care for the young chronic sick. She will continue visiting particularly difficult cases and give you feedback on how they are managing at home.

Visitors/relatives

I think the problem of communicating with relatives probably worries the newly qualified Staff Nurse more than any other area. As Jenny Dale said in her introduction: 'Their endless questions frightened me. How much of what I knew should I tell them? Was it my duty to do so?' There several golden rules regarding what to say and when to say it. There is also an awfully large grey area where what you say depends on how you feel as an individual exercising her professional judgement in a given situation.

I feel it is necessary to inspire confidence. If you are asked a question to which you honestly do not know the answer it is not enough to state boldly 'I don't know'. Honesty is admirable but it can be interpreted as indifference or even incompetence unless qualified. For example:

Relative: 'Staff Nurse, my mother seems to be in a lot of pain. What is wrong with her?'

Staff Nurse A: 'Oh, er – yes, she does, doesn't she? Well, we don't really know what's wrong with her. She might have had a heart attack. I'll tell the doctor you want to see him...'. Thankfully answers ringing 'phone.

Staff Nurse B: I'm sorry your mother is in pain. She has just had an injection which will soon make her more comfortable. As yet we really have no proof as to the cause of the pain but from the history it sounds as if she might have had a heart attack. We have taken a reading of her heart but that doesn't show anything conclusive. We'll be keeping her in for observation and we may learn more from some blood tests we'll be taking over the next few days. We'll let you know when we find anything definite. Meanwhile we just want her to rest and we'll be keeping a close eye on her. Could you just wait a minute while I answer this 'phone?...'.

You are reassuring the relative that you know of his mother's discomfort and have done something about it. You are taking measures to find the cause. You will keep him in touch. Most of all you have got time for him and if you have time for the relative you are bound to have time for the patient. That is one of your golden rules: you must always seem as if you have all the time in the world to answer questions even when you know you have a million and one things to do.

If a relative asks a question such as 'How long will he be in?', you are bound to be able to give *some* idea. Fill in as much as you can. It might be: 'Well, it rather depends what we find when we operate. We really can't say until then but it will be at least a week after surgery and may be longer. We will be able to give you a better idea after the operation.' Or, for someone who has had a cerebrovascular accident: 'Well, we can't let him come home until he can manage safely. He goes down to the gym every day and he's working very hard – just encourage him to do his exercises. Would you like to come and work with the physiotherapist one day to see how to transfer him, and when you feel confident you can take him home one Saturday and see how you get on.'

Visitors rightly expect you to know what's going on. You must use your judgement as to how much of what the doctors suspect you will tell them. The million dollar question is always 'Is it cancer?' If the patient has just arrived and you know the diagnosis is 'query carcinoma' you can honestly say 'We can't rule that out but there are lots of other things it could be and we'll be doing tests in the next few days to find out'. I would be reluctant to mention the word 'cancer' myself without absolute histological proof that I had seen with my own eyes. I am sure we have all admitted patients with a diagnosis of '? ca' made on X-ray which turns out to be totally unsubstantiated when the X-ray is seen by expert eyes. So another golden rule is caution unless you are absolutely sure of your facts.

When it comes to telling relatives of a certain diagnosis of cancer the task usually falls to the doctor. It is then vital that you find out exactly what he has said and how black a picture he has painted so that you have got your facts straight when you in turn have to deal with the relatives. For example, when a young man presents with Hodgkin's disease, which has been diagnosed early and will be treated promptly, the prognosis is very good and no-one must be left in any doubt about this, whereas a patient presenting late with lung cancer and cerebral secondaries will have a poor prognosis. In this case your approach must be equally positive but along the lines of pain relief and support to keep him at home as long as possible (if this is what he wants) with the ready possibility of terminal care in a hospital or hospice, if this becomes necessary.

While being positive, I make another golden rule not to be too optimistic when dealing with close relatives in privacy. I would always prefer to prepare people for the worst so that they are relieved when it doesn't happen. For example, following admission after a sizeable cerebrovascular accident or myocardial infarction, I may point out that, yes, things seem stable at the moment but the next few days will be critical and we will be observing the patient very closely. Likewise, while I am sure there is no need to itemize every complication of a given operation, if the patient is to undergo major surgery his relatives should not be led to think it is a simple matter of a few snips and sutures, or they will get a dreadful shock when they come to visit on the first post-operative day.

If relatives at any time express a desire to talk to the doctor, do everything possible to arrange this. In the first instance they may wish to see the House Officer, Senior House Officer or Registrar. This may be possible straightaway. If not, make an arrangement for the future remembering that, even when forewarned, doctors cannot always be certain to be free at a given time. If the interview can be arranged during visiting time there is more leeway. If the relatives wish to see the Consultant this may be possible before or after a ward round. Alternatively you may have to contact the Consultant's secretary to arrange an appointment. Some relatives never express the wish to see a doctor – it is part of your role now to decide when relatives (usually those of a critically ill patient) need to be seen and to suggest and arrange an interview. It is helpful to make a note in the Kardex of when relatives have been seen. On the other hand, some relatives wish to see the doctor daily. It is then your place to explain that there have been no developments, to talk to them yourself and reassure them that as soon as anything is discovered they will be informed.

Answering the telephone is another great worry. The first rule is to make sure who you are talking to before you say anything at all. If a close relative is on the line, especially someone you have spoken to already and feel you know, you may be able to speak quite freely. To be told a relative is 'stable' or 'satisfactory' may be reassuring but is not particularly enlightening. If you say 'She slept well for most of the night and has just had a boiled egg for breakfast. She would like us to wash her hair this afternoon', you are not releasing confidential information and yet you have said so much more. Remember always to pass on 'phone messages, however simple. If the enquiry is a distant relative or friend, innocuous information may be given. It does no harm to say that someone is 'comfortable' or 'in for a few tests'. If people want to know more they should contact the close family. If the enquirer is an employer I usually check with the patient first before saying anything at all. With the patient's permission you might be able to give some idea of the length of stay. You certainly need not give any details of the illness.

When close relatives ask difficult questions over the 'phone they should be encouraged to come to the ward. When you are face to face you can see whether you are being understood. Over the telephone words are easily misheard or misinterpreted.

Bereavement is always a difficult subject to tackle. There are any number of books to consult (for example, Kübler-Ross *On Death and Dying*). In simple terms the longer you have to prepare someone for an imminent bereavement the easier it is to tell them when death occurs – not just because they are prepared but because in talking to the relatives over a number of days or even weeks you have come to know them. The days are gone when nurses were expected to be totally unmoved by the death of a patient. Personally, I find the more in control the relatives are, the more moved I am – the more hysterical the relatives, the more I feel the need for control and calmness. If the relatives have had a long vigil, providing someone is there to take them home, they are best away as soon as possible. They might like a few minutes alone with their relative but are best not left too long. They may need reassurance that they were not to blame for the death, by for example telling them that they could not have predicted it would happen, or even if they had brought him to hospital sooner nothing more could have been done. Make sure someone knows where to come for the property and death certificate; if possible give written instructions which can be referred to later. Ministers of religion are often very comforting to relatives and will sometimes take them home.

If someone is suddenly taken ill make sure you know which relative to 'phone first. There is no point contacting a disabled husband and telling him to come immediately if he has no means of transport. Again, make quite sure you are talking to the right person before you give your message. If there is no telephone number a police message can be sent via the local police station but this is a very upsetting experience. You begin to understand why it is so vital to have the telephone number of more than one relative if possible or the number of a neighbour or friend who can pass on a message in an emergency.

It is unfortunately sometimes necessary to tell someone of their relative's death over the 'phone. Unpleasant though this is, I personally see no point whatsoever in making someone rush up to the hospital, heart in mouth, having been told their relative is critically ill when you know perfectly well he has died. It is never easy to break such news; there is no kind way of proceeding. From personal experience I would say it is best to state clearly and fairly concisely what has happened rather than trying to break the news gently. They can tell from your voice that something serious has happened and the suspense is dreadful for them if you hover and hesitate, unwilling to upset them. You must first establish beyond all doubt that you have the right person. For example: 'Hello, is that Mrs Smith of 4 Carlton Gardens?' 'Yes'. 'Your father, Mr David Jones, is a patient on Ward 6 at the City Hospital?' 'Yes'. You then go on to identify yourself and tell them what has happened. If you know they are not alone the task is very much easier for it is virtually impossible to comfort someone over the telephone. I usually say something like this: 'I am sorry to have to tell you that your father has just collapsed at the hospital and although the doctors did everything that was possible, I'm afraid he has died.' I know it sounds horrible. Once you have broken the news it is vital to keep talking. After the initial shock they will want to know exactly what happened. They might be comforted to know that the collapse came out of the blue – 'He had just finished eating his tea' or 'He was sitting reading his newspaper, he can't have known anything about it'. Reassure them that he did not suffer, that everything was done to save him, that no-one could have predicted what would happen. These days people often prefer not to come and see their relative when bereaved but you must tactfully find out whether or not they wish to come, so you know whether to lay the body out or not. You must also give the details of when and where to come for the certificate and belongings. It is thankfully often possible to sort out the practical details with someone else.

In the case of a death which is half expected and yet the relatives are not present the emphasis should be on the peacefulness of the death, if possible. 'He didn't seem to be in any pain'; 'He simply died in his sleep'; 'Nurse was with him when he just stopped breathing'. The more comforting information you can give the better.

Incidentally, there may be complications of the family tree – children from two marriages, for example – so that two or three 'phone calls are necessary before everyone has been informed. The legal next of kin should be contacted first.

Conclusion

As you can see, the role of the Staff Nurse is multi-faceted; being 'all things to all men' just about sums it up. Preparation is difficult. Ward management teaching in Schools of Nursing is helpful in that it stimulates thought and airs some of the problems. Most third-year students find their management assessment a useful exercise in starting to learn how to run the ward. It is helpful if finalists can have 'in charge' experience while a more senior member of staff is present to advise and support them. In practice, this is only possible when the ward is well staffed so the trained member of staff is virtually supernumerary. A defined period on a ward as a 'pre-registration Staff Nurse' with full recognition of the imminent change of status would surely be useful.

Most third-year students, if they are honest, feel ready to accept more responsibility. They see ward management as a challenge. The 'real' Staff Nurse cannot be created in the library or the classroom but can only begin to develop on the ward. Passing your finals is really rather like passing your driving test—an unpleasant necessity after which you are licensed to practise alone. Unlike the driver, however, you are surrounded by people who can help, advise and support you – make the most of them!

Further reading

Charles-Edwards, A. (1983) *The Nursing Care of the Dying Patient.* Beaconsfield Publishers.

Kübler-Ross, E. (1970) *On Death and Dying.* Tavistock Publications.

Kübler-Ross, E. (1975) *Death – The Final Stage of Growth.* Spectrum Books, Prentice-Hall.

Matthews, A. (1982) *In Charge of the Ward.* Blackwell Scientific. (Although intended primarily for Ward Sisters and Charge Nurses, this book gives lots of useful and thought-provoking advice for any nurse.)

Parkes, C.M. (1975) *Bereavement – Studies of Grief in Adult Life.* Penguin.

The Staff Nurse and Learners

Susan Cottam

You have passed. However, this is not the end of your education but a stage in your professional development. Think first of all how much success has changed your responsibilities. You are now not only a nurse but about to become a manager and a credible teacher as well. I say 'credible teacher' because all nurses teach each other even as junior learners, whether consciously or subconsciously, but now that the official letters, RGN, are after your name here is proof that you really do know what you are talking about. 'Well, Staff Nurse says...'.

It is the alteration in responsibility which is the first and most important role change. Responsibility towards the patient is one of professional and legal accountability (see chapter 5) not only for the care prescribed and given by you but also for the care given by other workers in your charge. The main group of workers will be the learners and the aim of their clinical allocation to the ward is to put the theoretical knowledge already learnt into practice and to build on it constructively. So what do learners expect from you?

Teaching

What should you teach them?

It is said we nurse with our head, hands and heart. Therefore there is need to:

1 Help learners to extend clinical knowledge so care may be planned intelligently, endeavouring at the same time to stimulate interest to find out more.

21

2 Help them to perfect manual dexterity in order that the art of giving care gently and skilfully may be acquired.

3 Always exhibit a caring attitude and teach the best way of delivering care with due regard for the patient's comfort, safety and dignity, so that patients can be nursed with consideration and empathy.

When and how should you teach them?

Most of your teaching will be by example. It often appears that nurses do not think that they can learn anything through any means other than listening to a formal lecture. It is difficult to realise that continuous learning is occurring sometimes consciously, sometimes subconsciously, by watching, listening and doing. Hazel Allen's book *The Ward Sister* highlights the fact that we learn from a role model. The oft quoted maxim that you remember some of what you read, more of what you see, but most of what you do, is well applied to nursing. A Staff Nurse is in a prime position to steer learning along constructive lines as she is the one with whom learners will be working most closely at the bedside. What a wealth of information and skill can be passed on to a learner! Imagine bed-bathing an unconscious patient. After a preliminary warning about an unconscious patient's hearing, and therefore the need to be careful about what is said, there is the opportunity whilst working together and clearing away afterwards to explain the rationale behind a multitude of nursing procedures.

Apart from demonstrating the actual technique of a skilful bed-bath you could explain why it is so important to maintain the integrity of the patient's skin, how this is done and the consequences if care is lacking, special points to bear in mind when performing mouth care on an unconscious person, the best way to take his temperature, how to position him and why, care of his joints and limbs and the reasons for doing passive leg exercises. The patient may need his airways aspirated and he may have a nasogastric tube in situ through which he is being hydrated and fed. The skills involved emphasize the importance of maintaining the patient's airway so that this point constantly recurs and is re-emphasized as being the most important consideration in nursing an unconscious patient. Even if this point is all the learner remembers the time spent will have been well worth while. The patient may also be catheterized and so the opportunity to teach the care of an indwelling catheter presents itself. The importance of noting bowel actions could naturally follow on.

As an adjunct to teaching, the learner may be asked to follow up some of the things discussed. For example, she could find out the signs of a deep vein thrombosis and then explain them the next time you work together.

These sorts of opportunities must not be missed as the chronic shortage of staff means that there is little time on today's busy wards for formal teaching. It is, after all, the practicalities of skilful bedside nursing which they have come to learn.

Schools of Nursing are now teaching principles so the learners are not taught a rigid set pattern for each nursing procedure. These principles of care can be adapted to suit individual patients in different circumstances and modified to suit the ward situation at that time whilst still following hospital policies. The Staff Nurse has an important part to play in helping learners to assess patients' needs and plan care in terms of priorities when there are pressures of time.

Time of course may not be the only thing lacking. Lack of supplies such as clean sheets and equipment (e.g. only one Ambulift) all serve to frustrate further, and when enthusiasm is blunted and ideals constantly undermined, it is so easy to become apathetic and indifferent. Somehow it is important to help them come to terms with the fact that nursing is not black and white but many ever-changing shades of grey, and adaptability is a quality which must be developed. There is no room for rigid thinking because the learner will constantly find herself having to rethink plans in such a constantly changing environment as a hospital ward.

Although the environment and ward situation may not always, if ever, be ideal, that should not prevent one aiming for the highest standards possible. This is all part of the challenge of nursing. When the learners have done their best to meet this challenge it is your support and guidance that will give a sense of satisfaction and achievement.

Another reason for making sure that no opportunity is wasted is that learners today get very little general experience due to so many specialized experience requirements. Therefore during their short stay with you they need to be shown particular points of nursing care which are relevant to the specialty of your ward, which may well not be found in generalized textbooks.

For example, learners will certainly be taught in school how to administer medicines in accordance with hospital regulations, and pharmacology books for nurses will explain how these drugs act. It may be difficult to find explanations of the finer points of drug administration, such as the reason for a Ventolin inhaler being given to the patient prior to a Becotide inhaler, when the two are prescribed to be taken at the same time, or how to make up a nebulizing solution. Many such points will be dictated by the policies of the physicians in charge and the advice of the hospital pharmacists.

It can be concluded therefore that Schools of Nursing and general textbooks may not be able to give specialist guidance in some clinical areas. So it's up to you again.

Apart from the conscious teaching that you do, whether formal or informal, just as some of the knowledge the student gains will be learnt subconsciously, so some of what you teach will occur in the same manner.

As discussed earlier, the learner gains knowledge by watching and listening and you may not always be aware that she is watching you or listening to what you say. Indeed she may not consciously realize this but gradually your overall attitude to work and to the patients will be assimilated and emulated. Do you genuinely seem to enjoy your work? Can she feel sure watching you that your position is what she eventually wants for herself?

How do you manage relatives? Is it obvious that you consider them important to the patient's overall well-being? Do you treat them with courtesy and respect, showing understanding and kindness during anxious times or does your manner portray that they are a nuisance? How do you handle difficult situations? Do you easily get flustered? Do you lose your temper quickly? Where do you place your priorities of care? Do you show that it is more important that the patients are comfortable and cared for than for all the beds to be made by 9 o'clock regardless of other priorities? How well are staff organized and co-ordinated when you are in charge: do they know what they are meant to be doing? Is there always someone around that they can turn to when they are unsure?

When everything seems to be going wrong can you still smile and see the funny side of things? Can you laugh at yourself? Everyone does foolish things occasionally. Learners will pick up your attitude to your colleagues. Are you loyal to them? How do you react to your seniors, the paramedical staff and the medical staff? Is it evident that you are sure of your own role amidst all these other professionals who are working towards the same goal? Is it obvious that you value your own worth in 'the order of things'?

The learner will react to your professional attitude. You are not just a teacher of clinical skills but a complete role model and, although some of these aspects will take time for you to assimilate and feel comfortable with, the point is that as far as the learners are concerned you are now Staff Nurse. The fact that you were still a student yourself only a short time ago is immaterial to them and not until they qualify will it be realized that adapting to these role changes does not happen overnight.

A learning situation which does recur methodically and without fail every day is the 'report' session or hand-over. It is an ideal opportunity to hear their assessments and care of their patients and discuss the nursing care plan. In order to make the report as helpful as possible there are a few points to bear in mind.

First of all, be specific. Don't just ask them to 'push fluids' for a patient. Vague statements like that achieve nothing. Give an amount to aim for. The same with observations: don't just ask to be informed if a patient's blood pressure falls – give a limit. Make sure they know what to look for when making observations of the patient and what must be reported.

Some information about the investigations ordered by the

medical staff and the aim of the treatment prescribed will help to increase understanding of the patient's overall management and highlight how the medical care and the nursing care complement each other. Other helpful information which will enable patients to be nursed more confidently will be whether or not a person is for resuscitation, especially when there might be reasonable doubt. If the illness has a poor prognosis it is important to know what information has been given to the patient and family. It is the learners that are the most heavily and closely involved with the patients and they are the most inexperienced when it comes to answering awkward questions.

One of the most unhelpful things when giving the report is to talk in abbreviations as there is little chance that the junior nurses will understand this code language. If the Ward Sister has made arrangements with other departments for the learners to watch investigations undertaken on the patients, then try to make sure that opportunities are not lost. Involvement with the investigation should give a better understanding of the importance of proper patient preparation, both physically and mentally. For example, in barium studies of the large bowel, if preparation of the bowel is inadequate the patient may well have to be subjected to the investigation again. This is not only distressing but a waste of the X-ray staff's time and repeated work for the nursing staff, besides being a cause of delay in diagnosing the patient's illness and therefore his treatment. It will also ensure that the need for any special precautions in the patient's aftercare are understood more clearly and may create more understanding when receiving the patient back on to the ward. Many procedures can be unpleasant and uncomfortable to someone who is ill. The knowledge of what happens to the patients when away from the ward and out of our hands will promote a spirit of enquiry into investigations for research purposes to which the patient has agreed but will not be of direct personal benefit.

On surgical wards it may sometimes be possible for the nurse to stay with the patient right through his operation. This may give added comfort to the patient and insight into his aftercare for the nurse. She will be able to visualize the length of the drainage tube inside the patient and will therefore understand the principles behind shortening and removal of the drain. Attending the out-patient department as an observer in a clinic also gives added insight into overall patient care, for example the problems medical and nursing staff face due to poor compliance in drug taking when treatment has to be continued at home. If this is due to poor understanding the nurse may be able to identify the specific problems and supply the information needed by the patient. However, non-compliance is a very complex problem and is not easily solved. Another advantage to be gained from attending the clinics is to observe conditions that are often treated in out-patients only. Myxoedema is one example (although this may involve in-patients if the patient is brought into hospital suffering from hypothermia, of which myxoedema may be an underlying cause).

The Nursing Process, used as a basis for care planning, is another teaching aid in itself. Learners can be guided to plan care systematically and objectively whilst adapting it to the individual patient. The Ward Sister will also expect you to help in explaining the application of the Nursing Process in your clinical area. Although principles remain the same, details of its practice vary in different areas. Using the admission assessment as an example, you may find that some medical Ward Sisters prefer the full assessment to take place over a period of time. If a patient has been admitted via Accident and Emergency, probably in pain or having difficulty with breathing, he will already have gone through one interrogation in Casualty with another one to come from the House Officer on the ward. However a certain amount of information is obviously necessary so the learners need to procure the immediately relevant details and continue to a complete assessment at a more appropriate time.

A surgical Ward Sister admitting patients to her ward for elective surgery may have a different policy as the patient may be for theatre the next day and information is needed straightaway.

I will not dwell further on the Nursing Process as it is

covered in chapters 4 and 5. However, learners need to know their objectives and the limits of their responsibilities. It is essential for all the qualified staff to share the same expectations of each learner in order to ensure continuity and consistency of ward experience, creating a harmonious atmosphere which is conducive to learning.

It is unsettling and confusing if, for example, one Staff Nurse allows them to do dressings and another doesn't, and similarly if you know that it is your Ward Sister's policy for a qualified nurse always to be present at the administration of drugs, then these wishes must be respected. One of the qualities which needs to be present if a good working team is to be created is loyalty to the leader and colleagues, and it is obviously much more pleasant to work as a member of such a team than one which is fragmented and disjointed.

The Ward Sister should inform you, on taking up your post, of aspects of ward and nursing management about which she has particularly strong views, such as the administration of drugs. It does not mean that she is necessarily set in her ways but that through experience she has learnt the safest and most practical way of managing the ward. Having definite policies will help put some structure into your role.

In order to help qualified staff share the same expectations of each learner, printed learning objectives which take into account various stages of training demonstrate quite clearly what should be accomplished during the allocation. These objectives will probably be given to the learner by Sister at a preliminary interview and you will need to be familiar with them to help the learner effectively. Once the learners have objectives the next problem is monitoring the achievement. The main means of assessment is a document arising from the King's Fund Report. This is given to the learner at the end of her allocation. Although it is customary for the Ward Sister to write and give this report she will no doubt turn to the qualified team for confirmation of her own assessment. If you find that a learner is not matching up to what is expected, mention it to Sister. She may feel that an intermediate interview will be beneficial and it might bring to light personal problems which may be hindering the learner's progress and which can be taken into account. Sister might also feel that a word with the learner's tutor is indicated. She will also know whether or not there have been problems with work on previous allocations. Some sort of useful information should transpire. Don't leave the problem too long before voicing your thoughts as the learner needs time to show improvement can be made. Few learners should get a 'bad' report unless of course they are totally unsuitable for nursing. It could be indicative of failure on the part of her teachers. Most nurses want to be thought of as good nurses so they should be given a fair chance to show their worth.

One other form of assessment carried out in the clinical area which causes a lot of anxiety for the learners is the ward-based practical assessments for the Roll and Register. The major cause of the anxiety, apart from natural examination apprehension, is the different requirements expected by individual assessors, not only in the practical skills being demonstrated, but also in the depth of knowledge relevant to the aspect of care being performed. If your Ward Sister is an assessor this makes things much more straightforward because you will know what she will expect of them and you will therefore know to what level to help them prepare.

If your post is in a hospital where continuing assessment of nurse trainees is practised, clear-cut guidelines will be required from your Ward Sister about your role. No doubt she will again turn to her qualified team for confirmation of her feelings and findings as she does when writing the ward reports. You may find yourself involved in actually helping to formulate the learners' objectives which will form the basis for continuing assessment.

On any hospital ward some formal teaching is required when the opportunity arises. The Ward Sister designates a certain area of care to each member of the qualified team. Sister may also ask you to bring in any interesting articles relevant to a patient on the ward at that time to pin up on an educational notice-board. It may be possible to devise a formal continuous teaching programme. Tutorials which may involve nurse tutors or clinical teachers may follow the hand-over report.

Just one point more concerning the learners' education: It is a good idea when chatting informally with the learners at break times to foster, particularly amongst the more senior nurses, an interest in their profession as a whole. You may find that you are just beginning to develop professional awareness yourself as throughout your training there are so many other priorities. Nurses do need to take an active interest in their profession and its development. Reading the nursing journals helps to keep one up to date with current changes and future plans. For example, an important issue at the time of writing is the Griffiths Report. If the learners bring up topics about which you don't feel equipped to talk knowledgeably, mention it to Sister, who may take the opportunity for discussion. Learners appreciate this sort of added interest being taken.

Before leaving the educational aspect of responsibility towards the learners you might like to consider the use of textbooks in preparing for examinations. Nurses link theoretical learning with patients they have nursed and it is important that the information and practice of nursing is correct in the clinical situation. Learners are our Staff Nurses of the future on whom we will be relying to maintain and develop professional standards.

Moral and personal support

Apart from teaching commitments another responsibility is to give encouragement and support when the learners face new and potentially distressing situations for the first time, such as a patient's death. Most come across death quite early in training and if it is known that this is the first time, introduction to the situation should be sensitive. On the first occasion just simply take them to look at the patient's body and explain the sequence of events to follow. Let them do last offices with an experienced nurse the next time the opportunity arises.

Giving a first injection is another hurdle to be crossed. It is of course the fear of hurting the patient that is the worry, but it should be emphasized that with practice skill can be developed so that it becomes gentle but as firm as possible. Learners will gain confidence if they do it again soon after the first attempt.

Praise is good, so even if learners have not made a very good job of doing something for the first time, pick out the bits done well instead of just criticizing so they don't have a sense of failure. It is useful to evaluate their performance; usually they are very self-critical and keenly aware of short-comings. Ask how their performance could be improved. If a learner cannot immediately see where her performance was lacking, direct her thoughts along constructive pathways. You may simply have to spell things out but give her a chance to see if there is a better way of doing it before offering constructive suggestions. At first learners are usually full of enthusiasm and high ideals and eager to learn. Care must be taken not to destroy these with destructive criticism, bearing in mind that they quickly become emotionally and physically tired. In dealing with learners remember that they all have lives outside the hospital and come from a variety of backgrounds, sometimes from a different race or culture. A mixed ward may have male and female learners allocated. Some will be young, some more mature, but all will be of different character, temperament and personality. They may be following a variety of courses. There may be nurses doing a degree course gaining clinical experience, students seconded from other areas such as mental handicap, those already qualified in one field of nursing and wanting to qualify in another, or qualified nurses doing an ENB course. Also there may be members of paramedical professions such as radiographers, not there to learn nursing procedures but to see how a ward functions, and pre-nursing students who are assessing the possibility of a career in nursing.

Many of them will be subject to different stress factors. For example, the younger ones may have left home for the first time and perhaps after being an only child a learner now finds herself living and sharing with many others. Some will have come straight from school with no experience or knowledge of hospital life apart from what they have seen on television. What is their image of nursing? They have never dealt with the public before and now they are sharing the responsibility of caring for sick people. They may see little of their friends due to conflicting duties and unsocial hours make it difficult to get home to their families or cultivate personal relationships. Even though they may be surrounded by people it is still possible for them to be very lonely and unhappy. This could manifest itself in the learner's inability to settle on the ward and in working closely with them you may be the first to suspect that something is wrong. If a relationship is built up with the learner it might be possible for her to talk to you and benefit from your ability to listen sympathetically and offer of practical help. It might be that a slight adjustment to off-duty is all that is required to give her a chance to sort out her problem. The more mature students have their worries, too. For example, children need care during school holidays, aged parents may need help, the husband may face redundancy, in addition to all the other responsibilities associated with running a home. Everyone has different needs, possibly complicated by various problems, in much the same way as the patients have.

The process of nursing is a logical thought sequence that can be applied by everyone to all the situations which they encounter. This tool is applied to the learners and called 'the Teaching Process'. Adapted in the same way as the Nursing Process is to patients, a systematic approach identifies the needs of the individual learner.

Some learners will have quieter rather than forceful personalities and as nurses usually choose nursing as a profession, they therefore share the responsibility for their education. The quieter ones will not push themselves forward when it comes to seeing and doing new things, especially in the early days. It is important therefore not to neglect them but to make sure that they do receive the same opportunities and stimulation until they develop more confidence. Knowing that people take an interest may make all the difference to the continued pursuit of the new nurse's chosen career.

In your early days as a Staff Nurse, don't be surprised if you find some of the learners' questions intimidating as they question the care you are prescribing. These will probably come mostly from the older students and the degree nurses. It does not mean that they are criticizing you, so don't become defensive. An older woman will possibly view life in a different light to you; experience alters one's outlook and the nurses are now taught to question and base their care on scientifically proven facts rather than on one person's preferences. This applies particularly to nurses with a degree or who are undertaking a degree in nursing as their critical faculties are well developed. If, however, you really do feel that they are questioning your clinical judgement, just remind yourself that you are the one who has passed the necessary exminations and proved perfectly capable and competent to nurse the sick. Bear in mind that you could be wrong and accept a good idea. However, it is you who are *legally accountable* for the patients' care so you do what is best in your judgement.

In a democratic team you do not have to take up a dogmatic or dictatorial attitude but if you feel that their suggestions would not be in the patients' best interests, explain your reasons, confident in the knowledge that you are the *qualified* nurse taking the responsibility. With practice it does get easier to lead without being domineering. This only comes as confidence increases and you become a member of the qualified team. This is where you should find your loyalty to your Ward Sister repaid by hers to you as you refer your problems to her.

After talking about the learners' expectations of the Staff Nurse, what do you expect from them? The answer is their loyalty and willingness to learn the art of patient care.

In order to cultivate this professional relationship there are certain things you should not do. First, don't ask them to do something beyond their capabilities. This is frightening for them. They may well learn something by being thrown in at the deep end but this may be to the patient's cost. Although heavily committed to a learner's education you are totally committed to the patient's care and comfort. You are accountable if anything goes wrong. Second, never make anyone feel foolish. When you are told something that is already known or insignificant accept it, otherwise they won't come and tell you anything else again and the next time it might be something you don't know and should. Third, if you do have to admonish them do not do it in front of the patients, other staff or anyone else; take them aside and speak to them in privacy. Last, if they ask you something you don't know, say so. Nurses who are on the receiving end of other people's expectations mistakenly feel they ought to know everything, which is an intolerable burden. Get them to go and find out the information and then come and tell you about it. We are all learning, all the time.

Eventually your status will be acknowledged. This acknowledgement cannot be demanded and the sort of things you will be respected for are clinical knowledge, competence and expertise, your caring attitude, the belief you have in yourself, your professionalism, and your integrity as a person.

Further reading

Allen, H. (1982) *The Ward Sister*. Baillière Tindall.

Thomson, B. and Bridge, W. (1981) *Teaching Patient Care. Guidance for the Practising Nurse*. HM&M.

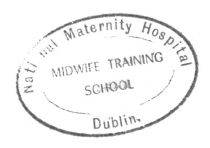

Relationships in Nursing

Lawrence Whyte

Relationships are connections or associations between or among people. The term 'interpersonal relationships' describes the relationships which are established between people and those with whom they come into contact on a one-to-one basis or in groups.

There is a shortage of written material on the subject of relationships within nursing. Whilst acknowledging that relationships as a topic cannot be taught or learned in the same way as subjects such as biology or anatomy, the limited written material applied to nursing practice is a problem. As an occupation, nursing inevitably involves working closely with people, whether they be staff or patients, for long periods of time. Most nurses would probably identify 'getting on with people' as a prominent and desirable aspect of professionalism. Teaching in interpersonal skills is not prominent in basic and post-basic nursing education.

When nurses discuss relationships it can be in a negative way. Within a hospital setting, for example, conversation may be directed towards the relationships among staff with little examination of one's personal values, beliefs or prejudices. This is sustained by the formation of several stereotyped images that are part of hospital life: the 'ogre' of the Ward Sister or the over-ambitious attitude of the senior nurses. The establishment of such stereotypes is useful for individuals in that they justify and reinforce the notion that, if there is conflict between nurses and their superiors, it is usually the fault of the superiors for it is they who cannot 'get on with people'. There is a myth that those who leave clinical areas have problems with relationships. Projecting blame on senior staff can deny the possibility of critical self-examination.

As a student nurse it is fair to assume that up until qualifying the relationships that you have experienced professionally have been transitory in nature between yourselves, your nurse colleagues and other Health Service personnel. These relationships have been constrained by the length of time that you have been allocated to a particular allocation, and by your relatively junior status up until now. As a qualified nurse you face the prospect of a post that will last considerably longer without the support and guidance you received from the School of Nursing and from your student peers. Just as the period following qualifying is a time to develop clinical, managerial and educative skills, so also is it a time to develop relationship skills.

It would be impossible to write a comprehensive or detailed account of 'how to get on with people' or to identify the characteristics that a nurse should possess in order to realize this desirable attribute with every patient or member of staff she ever encounters. If these things could be done, if it were possible to generalize about the subject of relationships, this would only serve to belie the fact that relationships are essentially individualized and unique between two, or a group of, people. Further, the characteristics of individuals that predispose the relationships that they have with others are dependent upon such variables as social class, development, values, beliefs and prejudices.

It is not the intention of this chapter to rely too heavily upon those areas of research or literature that have explored the subject of relationships, such as social psychology or interpretive sociology. Instead the approach of this chapter will be based upon the practical experiences or the anxieties and fears that the newly qualified nurse may encounter in the transition from student nurse to Staff Nurse.

Inevitably there are assumptions to be made in relation to this information. First and foremost is the assumption that, following qualifying, most nurses will be employed within hospital settings. Second will be the assumption that the problems identified will be pertinent to all ward settings when in fact individual wards and certain specialties, such as psychiatry, have paid a great deal more attention to the area of relationships, particularly staff relationships, than others. Third is the assumption that following qualifying all newly qualified staff are homogeneous, or at the same stage of development, when this is not true.Factors such as age, social background, personality and culture will influence the ability of some individuals to cope better in this transitional stage than others.

As nurses, we often use adjectives such as good and bad, which are relative interpretations, to describe relationships we have with other people. The factors that one person may identify as being conducive to a good relationship may be very different from the factors identified by another person. However, what is generally true is that certain conditions have to exist that contribute or make more likely the establishment and maintenance of a relationship that is mutually beneficial to the individuals concerned. Another problem in the professional relationship, such as that between a nurse and the patient, is that factors that could be identified as conducive to good relationships may not be equated necessarily with factors that are beneficial to those involved. For example, it may be unhelpful for a patient and nurse to have what might be described as a good relationship if this encourages the patient to become too dependent upon the nurse, or the hospital, or if the patient feels deterred from expressing hostile or aggressive emotions for fear of offending the nurse.

Working on the premise that relationships between staff ultimately affect and influence relationships with patients, I will deal with the former first. At the outset though, it should be emphasized that fostering and maintaining 'sound' working relationships is a reciprocal process. This chapter may be beneficial in terms of your approach to relationships but it is as well not to assume that the other people in the situation will automatically reciprocate.

Health care provision

The provision of hospital-based health care is team based and multidisciplinary in nature. No one occupation fulfils the entire need of one patient; rather, each contributes to the overall treatment and care. Without doubt there has been an enormous increase of professions and occupations engaged in providing some aspect of health care delivery. This is evident by merely looking at the services that are available to patients whilst they are in hospital: doctors, nurses, physiotherapists, occupational therapists, dietitians, radiographers, technicians, administrators, social workers and many others. All these professions and occupations are catering for specific needs of patients that provide a comprehensive service. This multidisciplinary nature of health care provision is team based because the objectives of all the members of the caring professions is to provide the best available service to the patient. Each profession and occupation is basically bound by the same ground rules that are regulated and formulated by a combination of their own professional bodies or statutory committees, the laws of the land, and the policies and practices laid down by the employing authority or training school. These rules have as their basic premise the notion that no harm should be brought to the patient in a deliberate or negligent act.

Superimposed upon this framework is the growth of specialization within medicine so that a patient who has been admitted to hospital for a specific complaint will, more often than not, be screened for other underlying deficiencies or dysfunctions. If abnormalities are found there will usually follow a referral to a specialist in another branch of medicine if the condition warrants further medical intervention. Furthermore, each occupational grouping has developed its own managerial and training structure to provide supervisory functions so that patients' lives are not endangered whilst essential learning can continue. The result of these developments in hospital-based health care provision is that, as a newly qualified Staff Nurse, you can most easily be viewed as a small but important cog in a big wheel.

During your years of training you will no doubt have received lectures, seminars and practical demonstrations from several of these occupational groups. There may have been occasions when you have worked jointly with them on the wards to provide a service to the patients. The question must now be posed as to how the relationship between yourselves and these other health care professionals has changed on obtaining your qualification, and what conditions are desirable for the fostering of sound working relationships in the interests of the patients under your care.

As a trained nurse these occupational groups will be approaching you for information and advice about patients. The gaining of your qualification and the wearing of the status of that qualification (e.g. uniform, belt or badge) will increase the expectations of these colleagues.

Chapters 2 and 3 of this book have already covered the expectations of others. Therefore the issue must now be to identify the social attributes that you should display in order to establish and maintain sound working relationships with your Health Service colleagues.

In the first instance the existence of rules and procedures governing patient treatment and care, particularly in relation to protection against harm being inflicted by negligence or by malice, is a predisposing condition for the establishment and maintenance of integrity. The concept of integrity when applied to the activities of the health care professions means that they act honestly and without corruption towards the goal of providing the best available treatment and care for the patient. Underlying this meaning is the acceptance that the individual concerned is acting in the interests of the patient. However, at times the exact rationale of the individual concerned may be difficult to determine. It can only be determined by asking, in a polite and appropriate manner, the individual responsible for that particular aspect of the treatment or care programme to explain the rationale behind it for it must be assumed that he is the expert in relation to that particular aspect of the patient's programme and that he has acted as he has in the interests of the patient. If though on receipt of the individual's explanation it is still suspected that the professional acted without integrity, then it is the duty of the nurse to report suspicions to immediate superiors. For overriding the mutual regard and respect of our professional colleagues' capabilities and judgements should be the safety and well-being of the patients.

Associated with the concept of integrity is the concept of

respect. Respect is the consideration felt towards a person or thing that has good qualities. It is important to accept that other health care professionals have had as extensive and intensive a training as yourselves and, in many cases, they may have had more. Therefore, provided that it is accepted that in the majority of instances they act with integrity, the work they do should be as highly valued as your own. There exists an inherent relationship between integrity and respect. In order to understand the integrity that other professionals demonstrate it is important to understand the rules and policies that govern their practice; whilst in order to value the work they perform for the benefit of patients you will need to be aware of the principles that underlie their practice. One of the most useful ways to gain this information is not only from books or from formal lectures but by approaching these other professionals at an appropriate time during their work with the patients you are nursing, and relate the work that they are doing to the overall treatment and care plan of the patient.

This has obvious benefits to you for by gaining an understanding of the work they perform and how it benefits patient care, not only are you increasing your own knowledge but you will in time be able to more speedily identify the appropriate criteria and procedures for calling in these professionals' skills in helping other patients in your care. Furthermore, you may also have an opportunity to increase your clinical skills. For example, in my experience most physiotherapists are often very willing to pass on information and teach basic skills that can be practically employed by the nurse in the course of patient care, such as breathing exercises, passive physiotherapy techniques or interaction games that occupational therapists use in the care of the mentally ill. However, it should be emphasized that this passing on of information must not override the boundaries of each other's work to such an extent that the patient may suffer or that one or other of the health care team acts unprofessionally. In other words, the willingness and permission to practise the basic skills of other professional groups must be mutually agreed and entail no risk to the patient. To venture too far into the boundaries of another colleague's clinical boundaries or to practise their skills without permission or instruction and supervision is unprofessional.

The twin concepts of integrity and respect are dependent on the ability of both parties to communicate effectively. Communication forms an integral part of every nurse's work. It is a process, a step by step progression of operations directed towards specific expected goals. Communication is the means we use to relate and share our thoughts, feelings, attitudes, needs, desires, pains, turmoils and crises to others. Few individuals have an innate ability to say the right thing at the right time on a consistent basis. For the majority of people the ability to communicate effectively is a learned process. It is learned through collaboration with others, through experience and through study. It is also developed through an understanding of one's self, i.e. self-awareness.

A variety of internal and external factors influence the manner in which the message we may wish to convey is sent, received and understood. Failure to be aware of these factors to a sufficient extent may result in the breakdown of the communication network. Barriers to communication are then erected and the existence of such barriers hinders the establishment of sound working relationships. It is possible to identify seven such barriers to communication, an awareness of which will contribute to establishing and maintaining effective communication networks with health care colleagues.

1 A person's values, beliefs and prejudices shape the transmission, reception and understanding of both verbal and non-verbal messages. If a person is insufficiently aware of their own values, beliefs and prejudices or those of the person to whom the message is conveyed, this will hinder effective communication between parties. For example, insufficient awareness of one's own values, beliefs and prejudices may result in inconsistencies in the message being sent and detract from the credibility of the sender. In ordinary language we suggest that people are 'two-faced' in that they communicate different perspectives on the

same piece of news to different people. For example, qualified staff sometimes convey different messages to other qualified staff than they do to learner nurses. This may reflect their own underlying values or beliefs that they hold about the role and importance of learner nurses.

2 Similarly, if an individual is aware of his own values, beliefs and prejudices, he may assume that the person whom he is addressing holds identical values, beliefs and prejudices. It is sometimes an example of ineffective communication when nurses who have entered the profession on what they consider a vocational basis fail to take account of the fact that other nurses have entered for entirely different reasons, e.g. humanitarian reasons, career prospects or because of a lack of opportunities in other work spheres. Divisions may occur because those who are vocational in their perception of work cannot effectively communicate with those others by adapting their approach in the transmission of messages. Thus there are often divisions in many hospitals along the lines of trained/untrained or conventionally trained versus university trained nurses. Of importance to nurses in their relationships with patients are the different values and beliefs that patients from ethnic minorities may hold as a result of their religious or cultural background. Similarly, the nurse should be aware that language may hold different meanings to different groups.

3 Failure to keep to the point of the message being communicated is another barrier to communication becoming effective. For the recipient to derive meaning from the message there is a responsibility for the sender to communicate with clarity and direction. Thus at ward hand-overs there may be a set pattern of communicating whereby the name, condition and diagnosis of the patient are all communicated at the onset before any report on changes is given. Certainly the implementation of care plans is one method whereby clarity and direction of messages can be formalized and aid development. How commonly, for example, is information lost because during a hand-over the nurse giving the report is interrupted by the telephone ringing or by various visitors.

4 Failure to focus on the sender or the message being sent may be the result of inattentive listening. Hence it is often the case that messages will be inadequately received because the nurse will not interrupt work to listen or pay close attention to the sender of the message. Even in the busiest times on the ward, it is important to stop your routine to listen to the message being conveyed. Otherwise important information may be lost.

5 The use of generalizations in the sending of messages will make it more likely that the message being sent will be misinterpreted. Instead of using adjectives such as 'good' and 'bad' or 'fair' it is more appropriate to be more accurate in descriptions if the sender wishes the message to be interpreted correctly. For example, when reporting on a patients' sleep, don't just say 'he slept well', try to accurately describe the time he went to bed, when and how his sleep was interrupted, and what time he rose.

6 Interpreting the message according to your own value system may lead the recipient of the message to jump to conclusions about what is actually being relayed. The striving for objectivity will be lost. For example, to conclude that a patient is not receiving enough visitors, when a message is passed on that they have not had visitors for a number of days, may be a reflection of your own value system that suggests that patients should have visitors every day, rather than an accurate interpretation of the message. Don't, for example, state your own personal opinions as fact, provide advice, or offer pat answers to problems.

7 Failure to maintain personal integrity will result in an unwillingness by others to communicate with you. The components of communication pertinent to personal integrity are those of withholding information, giving misinformation or over-elaborating the message received. These tactics may result in other parties feeling that they are unable to communicate effectively with you because the respect they have towards you will be diminished.

Within this section the approach has been to demonstrate the importance and the interplay of respect, integrity and effective communication in establishing and maintaining sound working relationships with your Health Service colleagues. The seven identified barriers to effective communication should be used to review and evaluate your own communication skills which are an essential part of any nurse's job. Some in-service training departments focus upon communication skills as a core component of staff development with the more advanced departments using experiential techniques to develop these skills amongst nurses.

The nursing team and relationships with patients

Whilst the newly qualified Staff Nurse can expect to have increased liaison and communication with other health care professionals, it is the ward-based nursing team that will be the focus of everyday relationships. The ward-based nursing team consists of any member of the staff engaging or performing in nursing duties even though such involvement does not necessarily entail direct contact with the patients. Members may range from and include senior nurse managers, clinical teachers, nurse learners, trained and untrained staff.

The components of maintaining and establishing sound working relationships with other health care professionals that have already been identified remain equally important in relationships with the ward-based nursing team – those of respect, integrity and an awareness of the barriers to effective communication. However, on the assumption that relationships between ward nursing staff have a more direct influence on relationships between nurses and patients, it seems logical to expand upon other factors that may come into play.

Each ward in which you will be sent to work as a permanent member of the staff will have its own approach to care. This need not be overt and it may not be written down, but it should be possible to identify it quite easily. The philosophy or pattern of care is basically the direction that nursing care has been chosen to take in this particular environment.

Theoretically three major patterns of care can be identified, each of which is dependent upon such factors as the prognosis of the patients and the length of stay of the patients in hospital.These two factors are important in determining the degree of custodial or therapeutic intervention that is appropriate to the client group. The first pattern of care is the custodial approach which involves the performance of essentially household tasks such as feeding, clothing, socializing and helping the patients to bed. It is founded upon the assumption that little more could, or indeed should, be done for the patients other than to make them as comfortable as possible and prevent them from coming to further harm or danger. Broadly it is a pattern of care that has been adopted quite successfully in the care of the elderly, the long-stay care of the mentally ill, and the mentally handicapped. Treatment programmes are minimal for those being cared for and are in some ways considered inappropriate for intensive therapeutic intervention. Given this assumption the quality of the nurse/patient relationship is likely to have fewer of the characteristics than that of a professional person to a client. It is more appropriate for the nurse to adopt a variety of roles that are outside her training. The nurse may be the only direct contact that the patient has with the world outside. The nurse may adopt the role of friend or confidante in the absence of a supportive social network that a patient who has been in hospital for a long period may have lost. Certainly it is more appropriate that the traditional hierarchies that exist within acute hospital settings are abandoned and that the ward environment takes on an impression of being 'homely'. Social interaction rather than therapeutic interaction would also be more prominent and, hopefully, there should exist an atmosphere of informality. Usually within such settings patients are encouraged to retain their own personal possessions and clothing to reinforce the atmosphere of informality and homeliness.

The medical intervention pattern of care is one that is highly supervised by the medical staff. The patient's difficulties are viewed as an abnormality in structure or function of the human body that can be overcome by some physical or biological intervention, which the medical staff are the only ones qualified to perform. The nursing staff's work is organized around that of the medical staff and is principally geared to serving as the agent of the medical staff in dealing with the patient. Interaction between nurses and patients can take on an impersonal quality for it can be expected that the patient remains passive and follows the orders and instructions that are relayed and formulated by doctors. As a pattern of care this was perhaps the dominant mode within most ward settings, particularly where the nature of the patient's illness or the medical intervention was rapid, such as in surgical wards.

However, this second pattern of care has been challenged quite strongly within the last two decades, not least by nurses who have increasingly perceived their role as being more than just subordinate. The most dominant pattern of care that exists within hospital settings has come to be that of 'therapeutic intervention'.The therapeutic intervention pattern of care encompasses familiar concepts such as comprehensive nursing and total patient care and, more recently, the Nursing process. The development of planned nursing involving identifying problems, setting objectives and evaluating outcomes has resulted, among other things, in a re-evaluation and adjustment of nurse/patient relationships.

Within the bounds of this chapter it is only possible to list quickly the adjustments that have increased in importance through therapeutic intervention. Those of you who are unfamiliar with the use of the Nursing Process should refer to chapter 5 and the books and articles given at the end of this chapter under 'Further reading'.

Adjustments in nurse/patient relationships that occur through therapeutic intervention

1 Patients come to be viewed as active participants in their treatment and care rather than as passive recipients. The patients' own motivational activity and their experiences of being in hospital become an integral component in their

treatment and care, and are considered to be beneficial for their recovery.

2 Interpersonal relationships between nurses and patients take on an added significance as every encounter the nurse has with a patient can be used to establish or maintain a nurse/patient relationship.

3 The basis of the nurse/patient relationship is perceived as contractual in nature with both parties responsible and bound by the contract. Usually the contract is formalized as a care plan.

4 The relationship ideally should be collaborative with the nurse and the patient working together to identify the needs of the patient and the services that can be provided for meeting those needs.

5 The relationship is directed with the clear statement of goals or objectives defined.

6 The relationship should be educational in that if the patient lacks the information about a situation or is not very self-directed, then health teaching by the nursing staff is seen as appropriate.

7 The nurse can expect to work independently from other health care professionals in some aspects of providing care. The degree of supervision by medical staff is reduced and decisions in relation to nursing care are made by nurses.

8 The relationship between nurses and patients is professionally rather than socially based. Many of the services provided by the nursing staff should be research-based to determine their effectiveness and efficiency. The patients' progress should be accurately described and documented.

Although there may be predominantly 'therapeutic intervention' patterns of care within ward settings in Britain, the expectations that the patient will hold should remain the same under whichever model of care is instituted wards. Under the therapeutic intervention pattern of care, however, these expectations will take on a more formalized dimension.

Confidentiality As a nurse there is an obligation to share information about the patient which may have a beneficial or detrimental effect upon the patient's recovery with other health care professionals. It is the responsibility of the nurse to ensure that the patient is aware of this. The patients may wish to impart information about themselves which they do not wish to be conveyed to other members of staff.

Acceptance means the conveying of a non-judgemental accepting attitude. In short, viewing the patients and accepting them for what they are, no matter how different their values, beliefs, cultural and ethnic traits may be from your own. Acceptance of another in this way communicates to the patient an acknowledgement of his individual worth. It is an attitude of positive recognition and underlies the philosophy of the Nursing Process in that it encourages the nurse to begin where the patient is and to make use of the patient's abilities to achieve his maximum potential.

Trust. The promotion of trust can be influenced by several factors. Consistency and reliability are essential. The nurse must aim to do what she says she will do. For example, to delay a request from a patient by saying 'I'll be back in a minute' and then failing to return will undermine the potential for the patient to develop trust in a nurse. Consistency in the performance of your duties will reinforce an essential component of trust-competence.

Empathy means the ability to put oneself in the position of the patient. Empathy permits the nurses to increase their understanding of patients' behaviour by allowing them to identify the feelings of the patients. It is of course possible to over-empathize with patients to the extent that the nurse may abandon her professional stance of objectivity by becoming too involved with some patients and thereby limiting her involvement with other patients.

Responsibility. The concept of responsibility is a reciprocal component in the nurse/patient relationship. Responsibility defined as the state of being accountable for one's actions is discussed in chapter 5. There is also a responsibility on the part of the patient. The Nursing Process for example is a problem-solving approach with the implicit assumption that both nurse and patient may identify and overcome the presenting problems. Each time a nurse does something for a patient that they can do for themselves, the nurse diminishes the degree of autonomy that belongs to the patient by mistakenly assuming too much responsibility. It is often more difficult to work with the patient than to do things for the patient as nurses have sometimes been taught that the latter is an essential component of care.

The termination of the nurse/patient relationship is the time to evaluate your performance. In the absence of any such evaluation existing within nursing, the onus is on self-evaluation. The following list of questions are those which are pertinent within the framework of establishment and maintenance of nurse/patient relationships given in this chapter. It is important to realize that every relationship you may have with a patient is a learning situation and that the components of relationship building, such as communication skills, gaining trust, being accepting, displaying consistency and responsibility, being empathic as part of the appropriate use of the Nursing Process (or any other form of therapeutic intervention) can be developed and refined. You have probably encountered nurses who seem to have an innate capacity to get on with people but it is the translation of this social capacity into meaningful and professional competence that is open to development and learning.

Check list for evaluating performance in nurse/patient relationships

1 Have the goals that were identified been reached?
2 What contribution have I and the other members of the nursing staff made to the overall recovery (stability) of the patient?
3 Has the patient reached a higher level of functioning through therapeutic intervention?
4 Was I successful in motivating the patient to become an active participant in his treatment and care?
5 Did the patient express confidence and trust in my competence and capabilities?

6 Have I successfully documented the care given to this patient to a level that is intelligible to another nurse on the ward?

7 Did the patient express that he had learned from his experience of being in hospital under my care?

8 Did I utilize the full services of the hospital in this patient's care?

9 Did I accept the patients for 'what they are' and show sufficient awareness of my own values, beliefs and prejudices so as not to allow these to influence the way that I cared for them?

10 What have I learned from this relationship?

Some thoughts on leadership

Just as the ability to 'get on with people' is an individual phenomenon, so too is the capacity for leadership. Within a group situation, which is what a ward-based nursing team represents, where people embark upon a joint project such as the nursing care of patients, there is a need for some form of leadership. Some leaders are appointed, such as Ward Sisters, and such appointments should follow a period where the individual has displayed qualities that are recognized as effective leadership traits.

There are three identifiable leadership styles: autocratic, democratic and laissez-faire. Autocratic leadership is excessive controlling: the imposition of the will of the leader on others. The autocratic leader makes decisions, demands support, evaluates others, and blocks other members from assuming the leadership role. Democratic leadership includes everyone in discussion and decision making and allows for the free expression of ideas and feelings in an open manner from all members involved. Democratic leadership deals with conflict in a problem-solving way and invites feedback from others. Laissez-faire leadership, on the other hand, displays a dramatic lack of involvement with excessive permissiveness.

Ideally, there is a need to display two out of the three styles of leadership within nursing: autocratic and democratic. The laissez-faire style is inappropriate in a ward situation where responsibility for others is the primary objective of those employed there. For example, in an emergency situation such as a fire or a cardiac arrest, there is clearly a need for autocratic leadership, for someone to take control of the situation and give quick and effective direction. However, in ward policy meetings or staff change-overs, then the more appropriate form of leadership is that of the democratic style. Thus one important quality of leadership within nursing is being able to recognize which style of leadership is appropriate to a particular situation and acting in that style.

Face the fact from an early stage in your career as a Staff Nurse that you may be forced to make decisions which may be unpopular with your fellow nurses. The first priority is to make decisions that are 'patient centred' over decisions that are 'staff centred'. For example, in the absence of the Ward Sister you may receive a request from a member of the nursing staff for a change in the off-duty. In your judgement the result of granting the request may be that the standard of nursing care would be reduced and that patients may suffer, so you refuse the request. This is patient-centred decision making. If you agree to the request and change the off-duty knowing that patient care may suffer, then this is representative of staff-centred decision making. As long as you have considered all the alternatives before making your decision and can offer the justification of making the decision along consistent lines, then the decision cannot be questioned. The role of leader in the ward situation is to follow the objectives and policies of the organization in which she is employed.

People in positions of leadership can tell you that it is idealistic to think that you can be an effective leader and remain popular at all times. Within a group situation some decisions are going to prove unpopular with some people but popular with others. You can't please all the people all the time. Alliances within a group are changing constantly. Similarly the group is usually subject to change in response to staff changes or allocation of learners. If for instance you are unpopular for some reason this is only likely to be for a temporary period.

Ideally one leads by example by maintaining the highest standards of nursing care that are possible, thereby letting others know what they should strive to achieve. Showing consistency in your work is important for your patients as well as for the other nursing staff on the ward. Imparting your knowledge and skills to others is an essential part of your role. In the times when you feel your popularity waning, seek the support of your peers and your Ward Sister, as it is their responsibility to ensure that you develop and to point out areas of your work that can be improved.

Above all, remember that your work is centred around the care of your patients and your responsibility is to make their comfort and safety during their stay in hospital your primary concern.

Further reading

Armstrong, D. (1983) The fabrication of nurse–patient relationships. *Social Science and Medicine* Vol. 17 (No. 8), pp. 457–460.
Friedson, E. (1970) *Professor of Medicine – A Study of the Sociology of Applied Knowledge.* Dodd-Mead.
Long, R. (1981) *Systematic Nursing Care.* Faber & Faber.
Stockwell, F. (1984) *The Unpopular Patient.* Croom Helm.

Nursing Practice and Accountability

June Gingell

The development of professional, accountable and autonomous practice is more assured when the leadership and the practitioners have full and knowledgeable commitment to the same ideal. Nursing can develop from illness care to health care in two ways:

1 The medical profession assumes direction for health promotive and illness preventive care and brings nursing along as an assisted function.
2 Nursing asserts legitimate leadership and autonomy in those areas and collaborates with the medical profession in a true team effort.

What is nursing? This is a question posed many times. A variety of definitions are available, some of which will be familiar. Florence Nightingale said the nurse's role was to put the patient in the best position for nature to act on him. Virginia Henderson says that 'the unique function of the nurse is to assist the individual, sick or well, in the performance of those activities contributing to health or its recovery, or to peaceful death, that he would perform unaided if he had the necessary strength, will or knowledge. And to do this in such a way as to help him gain independence as rapidly as possible.'

What do you define nursing as? You have spent three/four years' training and you must now function as a qualified member of not only a nursing team but a total health care team. As a qualified member of the health authority you are responsible for educating learners, following district policy and, most importantly, organizing and giving nursing care.

The International Council of Nurses' code of ethics states: 'The fundamental responsibility of the nurse is four-fold: to promote health, to prevent illness, to restore health, and to alleviate suffering. The need for nursing is universal. Inherent in nursing is respect for life, dignity and rights of man. It is unrestricted by considerations of nationality, race, creed, colour, age, sex, politics or social status. Nurses render health services to the individual, the family and the community and co-ordinate their services with those of related groups.'

With regard to nurses and practice the ICN defines four major areas of responsibility:

1 The nurse maintains the highest standards of nursing care possible within the reality of a specific situation.
2 The nurse carries personal responsibility for nursing practice and for maintaining competence by continual learning.
3 The nurse uses judgement in relation to individual competence when accepting and delegating responsibilities.
4 The nurse, when acting in a professional capacity, should at all times maintain standards of personal conduct which reflects credit upon the profession.

During your training there will have been various experiences with regard to the provision of individualized patient care both educationally and practically. You will have your own thoughts and ideas on how it works and if it works. As a registered nurse you are in a position of responsibility to provide care based on the individual needs of the patient. This is in line with the UKCC and EEC educational directives for nursing which consider the needs for the learner to work in an environment of planned care.

Our own professional body, the Royal College of Nursing, which many of us look to for guidance and support, also stresses this point in its discussion document 'Standards of Nursing Care': 'Purposeful behaviour includes a specific cycle of nursing behaviour which can be observed to be goal directed. This cycle starts with a systematic and focused care which implies a continuous and dynamic pattern of assessment, planning, action and reviews.'

The present philosophy of the National Health Service is that 'the weight of responsibility for his own state of health lies on the shoulders of the individual himself' (DHSS 1976). If this is what is expected of the patient, professionals must provide him with the environment where he is an equal member if not chairman of a team set up to solve his problems. He cannot be in control if he is expected to behave as an item on a production line.

As a qualified member of the nursing team you must know what you understand by nursing. You are accountable for your decisions as well as your actions. This means you are liable to be called to account for your actions not only to the hierarchy and doctor as we believed in the past but to the patient, to other disciplines, to yourself, to your profession and to society as a whole. You are contractually obliged to do what is best for your patient based on an assessment of needs of nursing care. This may mean being in conflict with other disciplines but you must follow what you believe to be good nursing practice. If the patient makes a claim against you he will succeed if the practice you follow is unacceptable according to the standards of other nurses, not other professions.

During the past ten years a great deal of attention has been given to define how nurses provide care. A growing awareness of the need to provide individualized care has seen a move away from the functional method of organizing care, with tasks allocated to nurses depending on seniority. The care given was fragmented and gradually team nursing became the norm, care being given by a team of nurses, with ideally the members being of different grades led by a qualified nurse. To enable individualized care to be given the use of the Nursing Process is advocated. This is a system of planning nursing care which has four stages. The way staff are organized at ward level is dependent on the grade and number of staff available. Regardless of what name is given to the method of work organization, if care has been well planned following a nursing assessment it is easier to give and more meaningful to the recipient. The four stages are:

1 *Assessment.* What is the patient's problem described in terms which are meaningful to all, including the patient?

2 *Planning*. What is it that the nurse together with the patient can do to solve or alleviate the defined problem? Describe carefully the strategy to be used.
3 *Implementation*. Act upon the plan.
4 *Evaluation*. Ask yourself and the patient – did the plan work? If not, why not? What changes do we need to make?

These four stages are continuous: there is no beginning or end – the process is cyclic. Nursing care has in the past been based on inadequate information, on assumptions based on a specific disease or disability. The patient was told what care he needed rather than asked; from your own experience you will realize the two are not always the same. This is not to say that we only give the care the patient says he needs but we must use our own professional judgement to guide the patient as necessary.

The problems experienced when implementing the Nursing Process have been created by nurses not understanding the basic concepts but implementing it in a 'cookbook' fashion. We now realize that the Nursing Process works for the patient's benefit only if the nurse uses it intelligently and realistically. The nurse must have the ability to use a problem-solving approach and requires certain skills which are taught as part of the curriculum in Schools of Nursing; also on a post-basic level as part of in-service training. Belated though this is it will help many staff who have been qualified for several years to understand the changing emphasis and philosophy of direct patient care.

According to Roy (1976), 'the reasons why nursing uses a problem solving based process are (1) a client centred goal for nursing and (2) the accountability of a profession as a scientific discipline which is service orientated'.

The ability to make a defensible decision is something nurses in general are only just learning to do as we accept we can no longer 'pass the buck'. 'A defensible decision is one that can be explained and whose every step can be recalled if necessary' (Bailey and Claus, 1975). It is obvious that the nursing process provides the clinical nurse with a framework for decision making about patient care.

If you are working in a hospital training learner nurses there is an obligation to educate them in the practicalities of planning patient care. This follows a statement from the educational policy of the General Nursing Council in 1977 which requires the learner to work in an environment of planned care using the nursing process. As already discussed, this was re-emphasized in 1984 when the United Kingdom Central Council replaced the General Nursing Council.

We have all at some time questioned the difference between theory and practice. If used sensibly the Nursing Process is a linchpin to help resolve some of those differences. The report of the Committee on Nursing had as its goal the production of practitioners capable of giving total care in any setting. We all have a responsibility to ensure this happens. Whenever change occurs people will feel threatened; they reject new ideas, because they experience fear. It is important therefore to provide opportunity for all staff to discuss change and its implications. Peer support at ward level is one way of survival against mounting problems.

Nursing must be accountable for the service it provides. Nurses must be able to define what activities they perform and how these activities affect society. How does nursing promote health? We can only demonstrate this by using a scientific approach to show that situations change by our intervention. This method of applying a problem-solving approach benefits the patient, the nurse, the profession, and therefore society as a whole. I will discuss briefly the stages of the Nursing Process concentrating on the practicalities of each of these stages.

Assessment

This is the initial stage of the Nursing Process and probably the most important. It allows the nurse to gather information and review the situation in order to identify a patient's problem. Assessment involves collecting information, organizing information and identifying a problem.

Information should be gathered from all sources. The most useful tool that nurses have is powers of observation. You must use these powers and develop them in junior colleagues, especially the learner nurse. The skills of observation and recall are difficult and come mainly through experience. The learner when performing a task may concentrate so hard on the task that she finds it difficult to continue the observation process. It is your responsibility to help the nurse to see the whole patient rather than the particular part she is dealing with. The information collected by observation is objective; it can be seen by all. Always describe what you see without drawing conclusions. Every time the nurse sees the patient she should be using her powers of observation to collect any new data.

Subjective information is what the patient tells you. Write it down as the patient says it – do not change the wording. This ensures all staff have the same knowledge about the patient. The words used to help us use the assessment stage of the process efficiently do disturb some nurses. They see 'interviewing' and 'examination' as very formal words, unnecessary in nursing, and certainly examinations as being the domain of doctors. Remember these are only words used to describe an action. Interview is defined only as a 'meeting between persons'. Examination is defined as an 'act of examining; enquiry into facts' and examine as 'inspect carefully'. It is not the words themselves that are important but how skills are used to elicit the correct information.

The interview with the patient should ideally be in a quiet, private place, although this is not always possible. The problem is that 'admitting' a patient at the bedside is the accepted norm, not the exception as it should be. If the patient is mobile you should be able to find a quiet spot somewhere on the ward. Nurses tend to try to collect all their information at the initial interview. It is important to be selective about the information needed at that time and the amount needed depending on the individual patient and his condition. The initial fact finding can take place over a period of several days providing that essential information is gathered as soon as possible. For example, it is important to gather essential information such as the patient's address and next of kin, how they may be contacted, and the patient's perception of his illness and his expectations.

If admitted for overnight stay following a minor operation on his nose and otherwise fit, the patient will quite rightly have strong objections to answering questions on how many stairs he has at home. The assessment must be relevant to the patient's needs.

Gathering information about a patient's daily life helps us to foresee how his present illness/disability will affect his life on returning home if this is relevant. It also helps us to plan our care allowing for as little disruption in his normal rountine as possible.

Beware the practicalities of working in an institutional setting. Do not ask the patient what time he likes his meals unless you inform him what mealtimes are whilst in hospital. It is your responsibility to ensure the patient is not offered something which cannot be provided. You are the person who will have to deal with the complaints from the patient.

Examination

This is the last stage of assessment. By this time you should have developed a relationship with your patient to ensure he is agreeable to you 'handling' him. Examination is usually spoken of in the context of medicine but nurses examine every day. The recording of blood pressure and pulse are part of our examination. The information regarding a wound, such as size and colour, are documented following examination. It is not intended for nurses to listen to heart and lungs as the majority of nurses do not have the knowledge or skill to understand the significance of what they hear. Palpation of a part of the body may be necessary. The midwife palpates the abdomens of pregnant women. The ward nurse may feel it necessary to palpate the abdomen of a patient who complains of inability to pass urine. The examination may also be used as a tool to show concern. Purely by palpating his abdomen the patient will realize you care and are aware of his problem.

It is extremely important when assessing a patient by observation or examination that you have a scheme to ensure you miss nothing. Some use a body system, others a head to toe approach. When information is collected it should be recorded in an objective way, e.g. 'wound on rt buttock 5cm long by 8cm wide. Hard and black with red edges all round'. This ensures the next person knows exactly what to look for and if any improvement or deterioration has occurred. Once you have gathered your information by all the means available, decide what you will do with it. How do you organize this information so that it will help plan care? Use what works best for you. If you are working in an area training learner nurses, be conversant with the teaching of the School of Nursing and use it to help the learner understand use the information collected.

The use of activities of daily living are in common use and the reader should refer to Virginia Henderson's *'The Nature of Nursing'* (1966) or Roper, Logan and Tierney's *'Learning to Use the Process of Nursing'* (1981) and *'The Elements of Nursing'* (1980). Henderson lists a person's needs as follows:

1 to breathe normally
2 to eat and drink adequately
3 to eliminate by all avenues of elimination
4 to move and maintain a desired postion
5 to sleep and rest
6 to dress and undress and select suitable clothing.
7 to maintain body temperature
8 to keep body clean and well groomed and to protect the integument
9 to avoid dangers in the environment
10 to communicate and express emotions, needs and fears
11 to worship according to faith or conform to concept of right and wrong
12 to work at something which gives a sense of accomplishment
13 to play and participate in recreation
14 to learn, discover or satisfy the curiosity.

The physical needs must be met before the higher needs can be met.

Abraham Maslow has also set out a hierarchy of needs in which the physical needs must be met before those of higher intellectual levels. His hierarchy is as follows:

1 physical needs – must be met for survival
2 safety and security needs – things that make the individual comfortable
3 love and belonging – to give and receive love
4 esteem needs – feeling good about oneself; pride
5 self-actualization needs to meet set goals.

Roy, in 1976, described an adaptation model; this states that nursing's goal is to promote man's adaptation in situations of health and illness. Every individual copes differently and as he is also a member of a family and community no two situations are the same. If a nurse is to help a patient adapt to the changes around him she must identify the individual's level of adaptation and define his difficulties so she may intervene and promote adaptation. When the information has been organized by whatever method you find suits you the care plan can be formulated by the nurse and patient together.

Planning

Planning care for the patient is the next step in the Nursing Process. Information has been collected and the patient's problems defined; you must now decide how these problems will be solved, by whom, and where and what means will be used to determine if the patient is progressing. The patient must be involved in setting priorities if he is able to participate. The nurse may be wasting her time if she does not ask the patient the all important question 'What do you think is your biggest problem?' You may be surprised at the answer.

One of the big problems with planning care is identifying priorities. This is obvious if the patient's airway is at risk but sometimes the decision is not so obvious. If you understand

Maslow's hierarchy of needs it gives you guidance on organizing problems: physical problems override needs at a higher level. Do not expect a learner to write a perfect care plan. Her lack of knowledge of disease processes and her lack of experience are great gaps in her ability to set priorities. A badly written care plan is like a badly written drug sheet; if it is not clear, concise and continually updated it is like a dangerous weapon in the wrong hands.

No two patients, even with the same medical diagnosis, will need exactly the same care. The patient having a hysterectomy at 25 will need different care from a woman of 65. The care plan should reflect this difference in need and every member of the nursing team should be able to give the care accordingly.

There has been a great deal of discussion on how to define 'a problem' and 'goal' etc. on the care plan. Remember the plan must be safe. A patient admitted for control of hypertension should have 4-hourly resting and standing blood pressure recorded. If you feel this needs writing on your plan, but there is a question in your mind if hypertension is a nursing problem, write it down for later discussion with your colleagues. If you believe the plan is safe, then time for discussion will help everybody learn. The care plan is something to be used retrospectively to demonstrate how we define and solve problems and how we can progress. Implementing change will not happen overnight and we must be very patient and support each other.

Implementation and evaluation

Change is taking place constantly and other disciplines put pressures on ward staff because of changes taking place in their own profession. Nurses have in the past accepted the extra workload to the detriment of nursing care but we are now questioning the reasons behind the shifting workload.

Remember when planning care that part of the nurse's role is to carry out specific medical instructions – giving prescribed drugs, etc. All this must be taken into account when you are looking at the practicalities of implementing the plan. You can only give the care your resources allow. It is important to discuss with your Nurse Manager if you feel you do not have the right quality or numbers of staff that your patients demand but, if no staff are forthcoming, then reorganizing and replanning are required.

The necessity for increasing staff has traditionally been because the ward is 'busy'. This is no longer acceptable. You have to define why the staff are needed. The care plans should enable you to estimate how many nurses of what grades are needed. Remember when calculating staff needs on a daily basis to take into account the patients' abilities and, in many cases, the relatives' involvement. The aim is to return the patient to his home if possible and therefore the relatives should be involved in his care plan and giving care.

If you cannot give prescribed care to patients you must determine why. If the patient has not achieved the set goal, was it because the goal was unrealistic? Was it because we failed to provide the right environment or resources? If so, was this because they were not used correctly or were not available? When documenting the evaluation we must be professional enough to state exactly why the patient has not reached the desired goal. Avoiding the evaluation of a nursing action which is not working is detrimental to the patient. It is senseless to continue the same course of action if it is known not to be working. Sometimes it is difficult to decide what will work and it is essential that all avenues are explored and more expert knowledge sought.

The nurse has at her disposal a certain amount of expert knowledge to help her write care plans in the form of research publications. A quantity of literature is available on common aspects of care, for example, Doreen Norton's classic work on pressure sores which has only recently begun to be widely applied in the setting of the nursing process.

Because you can be called to account for any decisions, you must be seen to demonstrate an awareness and use of research findings to help plan care. Many research reports do tend to be off-putting but it is your responsibility to be aware of new thinking and ideas. Clark and Hockey (1979) wrote of the implication of research findings: 'To make use of research does not necessarily mean to implement findings – the use of research implies the reading of research reports with insight and comprehension in the first place – sometimes it will encourage the reader to pursue some of the references – sometimes the reader may simply be directed to situations which warrant special attention.'

It is not my intention in this discussion on the Nursing Process to tell you what it is or how to implement it but to discuss some of the practical problems that Staff Nurses have asked my advice on over the last few years. Remember, you are a member of a team caring for the patient to help him return to his normal state of health, or as nearly as possible.

At the beginning of this chapter I discussed briefly how we have progressed from a functional, traditional style of nursing. The nursing hierarchy is also changing from the mechanistic system of management adopted with Salmon to an organic system with decisions being made at levels where expert knowledge is available. This move puts even greater pressure on the trained nurse at ward level. She is expected to assess needs and plan care for her patients as well as give them care. She is also now being spoken of as a practitioner in her own right, a term previously reserved for midwives. In an effort to help nurses fulfil all the functions expected of them and ensure professional development, there is a significant change in the organization of nursing care/delivery system – primary nursing.

Primary nursing was originally organized to decentralize decision making and give maximum accountability to each qualified nurse. The registered nurse accepts professional accountability for the care of the patient in the same way that the physician does, throughout the patient's length of stay in hospital. A second nurse works with the primary nurse and patient to make up the team.

The primary nurse makes the decisions about care and communicates them verbally and through the use of the care plan. The direct communication ensures continuity of care. Other disciplines learn which nurse is responsible for the patient and communicate directly with her.

Primary nursing is a great challenge to nurses, with rewarding results. If given the chance you must ask yourself certain questions:

1 Would you feel prepared to accept total responsibility for patient care from admission to discharge?
2 How would you see your relationship with the Sister and Charge Nurse?
3 Would you be prepared to argue the case for certain nursing actions as opposed to those put forward by other disciplines?
4 Is the profession as a whole ready for this method of organization?
5 What financial implications are there for such a system? Are you prepared for the changes which are taking place in nursing which affect you at ward level?

In the past we believed that change affected the nursing hierarchy only but this situation no longer exists. All changes affect the clinical nurse in some way or other and we must be aware and prepared for them. After reading this chapter you may feel frustrated – few, if any, of your questions may have been answered. The intention is that you are aware of the position you are in and the responsibility you have to be prepared to take before any changes take place. I hope you will find help by reading some of the suggested books and continue to keep yourself up to date for the benefit of your patients and your own professional development.

References

Bailey, J.T. and Claus, K.E. (1975) *Decision Making in Nursing.* Mosby.

Clark, J.M. and Hockey, L. (1979) *Research for Nursing: A guide for the Enquiring Nurse.* HM&M.

Department of Health and Social Security (1976) *Prevention and Health: Everybody's Business. A Reassessment of Public and Personal Health.* HMSO.

General Nursing Council (1977) *Briggs Report of the Committee on Nursing.* HMSO.

Henderson, V. (1966) *The Nature of Nursing.*

Henderson, V. (1969) *Basic Principles of Nursing Care*. International Council of Nurses.

International Council of Nurses (1973) *Code for Nurses: Ethical Concepts Applied to Nursing*.

Maslow, A.H. (1968) *Towards a Psychology of Being* (2nd ed). Van Nostrand.

Norton, D., MacLaren, R. and Exton-Smith, A.N. (1975) *An Investigation of Geriatric Nursing Problems in Hospital*, p. 197. Churchill Livingstone.

Roper, N., Logan, W.W. and Tierney, A.J. (1980) *The Elements of Nursing*. Churchill Livingstone.

Roper, N., Logan, W.W. and Tierney, A.J. (1981) *Learning to Use the Process of Nursing*. Churchill Livingstone.

Roy, C. (1976) *Introduction to Nursing: an Adaptation Model*. Prentice-Hall.

Roy, C. and Roberts, S.L. (1981) *Theory Construction in Nursing: an Adaptation Model*. Prentice-Hall.

Royal College of Nursing (1980) *Standards of Nursing Care: a Discussion Document*. RCN.

Further reading

Clarke, M. (1983) *Practical Nursing*, 13th ed. Baillière Tindall.

Kratz, C.R. (1979) *The Nursing Process*. Baillière Tindall.

Mayers, M.C. (1976) *A Systematic Approach to the Nursing Care Plan*. New York: Appleton-Century-Crofts.

McFarlane, J. and Castledine, G. (1982) *A Guide to the Practice of Nursing Using the Nursing Process*. London: Mosby.

Pyne, R.H. (1981) *Professional Discipline in Nursing; Theory and Practice*. Blackwell Scientific.

West, A. (1980) Patient into person. *Nursing Mirror*, Vol. 150 (No. 8).

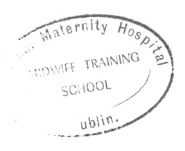

The Law and Nursing

Mia Telford

The need to study law and ethics is not always apparent to students of nursing. It is an area that is seldom explored. Yet law is a discipline that impinges on everyone's life by virtue of its real impact or its perceived threat.

The law seeks to protect the rights of one party against infringement by another. It may not always work in ways that seem just and when resorted to it will only administer the requisite legal rules with little recourse to the fairness of the situation. In many ways it is an unwieldy system and slow to adjust to social change. But at least it gives some order and stability to society.

With the development of health care services and the increased expectations that the public have of the National Health Service, aggrieved patients and relatives are now more likely to look for somebody on whom to vent their grief and frustration than when medical sciences had little impact on the course of a person's life, and when it was the same person who delivered all that care – usually the family doctor. In many ways the NHS has become the victim of its own success and if patients feel that they have been mistreated they know that they can look for a remedy in the courts.

Contemporary law has evolved from two sources – *statutory law* from Acts of Parliament and *common law* from judicial decisions. Statutory law usually arises because of social change and the need to modify that change while at the same time striving to uphold the social order. It is law written by Parliament and is a rigid system in that it lays down rules and regulations, and a breach of these rules for whatever reason usually constitutes a legal wrongdoing. Common law is the result of a series of cases brought before the courts for adjudication. It is more flexible than statutory law and is used to interpret and modify Acts of Parliament.

These sources can be split into two parts – *criminal law* which deals with actions which are an offence against the State, although they may have been aimed at individuals, and *civil law* which deals with one individual's rights against another (such as the law of tort or contract). Sometimes there is an overlap in that assault and battery are both crimes and torts, and a defendant may be tried in a criminal court but have damages awarded against him in a civil court.

There are two ways in which a nurse will encounter the law during the course of her work. Firstly, as an employee she should be aware of employment law, and secondly, as a provider of nursing care she should be aware of the law of tort and of criminal law.

The nurse as an employee

A nurse is employed under a 'contract *of* services'. This makes her immediately accountable to her superiors and they in turn direct the performance of her work. This differs from consultant medical staff who are employed under a 'contract *for* services' which allows them clinical freedom in that no-one can direct them in matters of clinical judgement. Most of the law concerning contracts of employment is now consolidated by the Employment Protection (Consolidation) Act 1978 which provides for written conditions of service and for minimum periods of notice.

As an employee the nurse acquires the rights and protection offered by the body of employment legislation. She cannot be dismissed either wrongfully or unfairly from her work. Wrongful dismissal is a breach of her contract of employment and is covered by the normal rules of contract and damages, whereas unfair dismissal is covered by the 1978 Employment Protection (Consolidation) Act. This applies to situations where people are dismissed without being given the appropriate warnings or because of trade union activities. Unfair dismissal also covers areas where the behaviour of the employer is such that it amounts to a breach of an express or implied term of the contract of employment. Unless the employee leaves soon after the conduct of which he complains he may be regarded as having elected to affirm the contract. Before anyone can claim unfair dismissal they must have been continuously employed for the minimum qualifying period of one year.

The length of time a nurse has served in one job is important because on that depends whether she is unfairly dismissed (1 year), the minimum amount of statutory notice she will be given, whether she will be entitled to a redundancy payment (2 years), whether she will receive maternity benefit (2 years), and the amount of any compensatory award. When an employee changes her employer she must start at the beginning again and build up time of employment, as years spent in previous employment are irrelevant for this purpose. But there are situations where a change of employer does not bring about a break in the term of employment, for example where an employee moves to an associated employer. If the employee's period of continuous employment is to include a period with a previous employer, the written statement of terms required by the Employment Protection (Consolidation) Act 1978 should include a clause to this effect. This could apply to health authorities within a Regional Health Authority but whether it would apply to areas in different regions is uncertain.

A nurse in employment is allowed reasonable time off work for trade union duties and activities. Where a nurse is a trade union official she is entitled to time off to undergo approved industrial relations training and to carry out official duties. These duties have been described in a Code of Practice issued by ACAS and include collective bargaining, explaining the role of the union to new employees, and appearing for members involved in industrial relations matters. The amount of time off varies according to the union's agreement with the employer. The official is also entitled to be paid for the time she spends on union duties, provided it is during a time when she would normally have worked – she is not entitled to overtime for union duties.

The employer is also obliged to allow members of an independent recognized trade union time off work during working hours for union activities, though not for industrial action. The amount of time spent away from work must not be unreasonable and should be determined in accordance with the ACAS Code of Practice. Unlike trade union officials, they cannot claim payment while absent from their duties. Where an employee is not allowed time off work for trade union activities she can present a complaint to an Industrial Tribunal but this must be done within three months.

If an employee who is a trade union official is dismissed or treated unfairly at work because of her trade union activities she, too, can complain to an Industrial Tribunal. If she can prove her case her employer may find himself paying her exemplary damages as he is not allowed to discriminate against an employee because she is a trade union official.

An employer cannot discriminate either directly or indirectly against a nurse on the grounds of sex or marital status, i.e. he cannot treat a female nurse less favourably than a male nurse, nor a married nurse less favourably than a single nurse. Nor can he unjustifiably apply a condition that would result in a small proportion of women being able to comply with that condition. There are a few exceptions to this which include working in a private household or where the nature of the job specifically calls for a man or a woman. The Sex Discrimination Act 1975 applies equally to men and to women, whether married or single, the only exception being that a man cannot make a complaint arising out of a special treatment given to a woman as a result of her being pregnant or because of her earlier retirement.

Similarly, an employer is prohibited by the Race Relations Act 1976 from treating one person less favourably than another by reason of his colour, race, and ethnic or national origin.

However, an employer also has expectations of his employee. These expectations can either be written into his contract as express terms or can be implied terms of contract. The employer will expect that his employee will be ready and willing to work, to offer personal service (i.e. to do the job himself and not ask or pay someone else to do his job), to take reasonable care in the exercise of his duty, and not wilfully to interrupt his employer's undertaking. He must also obey reasonable orders and be trustworthy and honest in his dealings with his employer.

Under the Health and Safety at Work\Act 1974 both the employer and the employee have specific duties. The employer must ensure as far as is reasonably practicable the health, safety and welfare at work of all his employees. This he does by the provision of plant and systems of work that are, so far as is reasonably practicable, safe and without risks to health. But it is the duty of every employee while at work to take reasonable care of his own health and that of others who may be affected by his acts or omissions at work. A nurse must always be aware of the possibility of danger to patients and colleagues and should report faulty equipment, unsafe floor coverings or anything that might constitute a risk to another. She should also ensure that her own practices are safe. When excluding air from syringes prior to giving injections, care should be taken that the contents are not squirted into the air and over everybody present, particularly when cytotoxic drugs are involved. If caring for patients with communicable diseases, the nurse must make sure that they are nursed in the manner appropriate to their particular infection and that others are not put at risk of contacting the organism.

It is a criminal offence to be in breach of the Health and Safety at Work Act. This Act only applies to property other than Crown property but hospital workers do not escape the protection of the Act, as the Health and Safety Executive will issue Crown Prohibition and Crown Improvement Notices as a means of getting health authorities to rectify any unsafe practices or equipment or buildings that might result in injury to an individual.

The nurse as a provider of nursing care

Those who fail to consider the legal or ethical implications of their actions all too often pay the price in terms of reputation,

71

happiness or money, but if behaviour is guided by ethical considerations, it is more likely to be legally defensible than if it occurs through expediency. An ethic is a standard of behaviour evolved over a period of time which reflects the principles that are important to a group. Ethics describe what ought to be rather than what is, they change as society evolves, and they cannot easily be ignored. Knowledge of one's own personal values within a professional code is vital if one is to be accountable for one's own actions and the consequences of one's own decisions. To this end the UKCC Code of Professional Conduct should be carefully studied and the nurse should keep abreast of any updating of the code. If a nurse commits an illegal act, whether she intended to or not, she will be indicted as a principal offender or as an accomplice, depending on the seriousness of her actions.

But when is a nurse likely to become involved with the *criminal* law during the course of her work? Perhaps the most likely occasion would be as a result of an assault and battery. Once a patient feels that your behaviour is going to result in immediate and unlawful violence to him, that patient has been assaulted, even though you have not laid a finger on him. Battery occurs once the patient has been struck. The amount of force used is irrelevant and the nurse does not need to have intended harm. Violence is not unlawful if a nurse is acting in self–defence, or if the defence of consent is available. Hence the importance of always obtaining a signed consent from the patient prior to operation.

Likewise, if a nurse commits an act in the knowledge that death will result, she may find herself open to a charge of murder or, depending on her intention and state of mind at the time, manslaughter. This is of particular importance when dealing with people on respirators who have not been certified as 'brain-dead' or where the usual formalities have not been completed. Nurses may also be charged in cases involving infants whose prospects of leading a full life are impaired, as happened recently when a paediatrician who gave a Down's syndrome child DF118 was charged with attempted murder, although he was eventually acquitted. There is no acceptable defence of euthanasia as this could lead to people committing murder with impunity.

Where a nurse is found guilty of a serious crime, particularly one where a patient is involved, not only will she be fined or imprisoned but she is also likely to lose her registration and with that her livelihood.

The area of law with which the nurse is most likely to come into conflict is that of tort. This deals with aspects of civil law and for a plaintiff (usually the patient) to succeed he need only prove his case on the balance of probabilities. (In criminal law, the state must prove guilt beyond all reasonable doubt.) A tort is a legal wrong which is independent of contract. The bulk of hospital legal problems are likely to fall within the tort of negligence.

The tort of *negligence* has only evolved within the last sixty years. Prior to that, to succeed a plaintiff had to show that he had a contract with the defendant – then along came the celebrated snail in the ginger-beer bottle! One evening in 1928 two Glaswegian ladies went into an ice-cream parlour and one bought her friend, Mrs Donoghue, an ice-cream and a bottle of ginger beer, half of which was poured over the ice-cream. When Mrs Donoghue had finished her ice-cream she poured the remainder of the beer, which was in an opaque bottle, into a glass and out popped the decomposing remains of a snail. When she saw this she was extremely upset, suffered nervous shock and spent some time in Glasgow Royal Infirmary with gastroenteritis. When she recovered she decided to seek damages but she could not recover anything from the owner of the cafe as she did not have a contract with him because her friend had bought the ginger beer. So she decided to sue the manufacturer of the beer, Mr Stevenson, because he had broken a general legal duty not to manufacture defective products. In his leading judgement, Lord Aitkin declared that the moral duty to love one's neighbour was to be incorporated into the law as a duty not to injure one's neighbour. For legal purposes a neighbour is anyone who is so directly affected by your conduct that you ought reasonably to have contemplated his being so affected.

For a negligence claim to succeed the plaintiff must show three elements:

1 that the defendant owed him a duty of care

73

2 that there was a breach of that duty of care
3 that as a result of that breach the plaintiff suffered damage.

If there is no damage then there can be no claim in negligence.

A duty of care is owed by a nurse to everyone who comes within her sphere of influence. Once a member of the public becomes a patient in hospital and in contact with the nurse she then owes that person a duty of care. The duty is owed to the plaintiff alone and not usually to others; it may be either an act or an omission which will constitute the breach. Where there is no duty of care there cannot be a breach unless you take steps voluntarily to involve yourself, so you can let a blind man wander over the edge of a cliff or leave an injured person at the scene of an accident in the care of unskilled hands secure in the knowledge that you will not be sued for negligence.

The required standard of care is that of a reasonable man. The test is that of a nurse who professes to have a special skill and exercises it. When looking at the standard of care the Court will consider how a fictitious nurse in the same circumstances would have behaved. Thus a Staff Nurse will be judged by the standards of a Staff Nurse and a Sister by those of a Sister.

If a patient is known to have a defect and harm results to him because of that defect, then he will have a case of negligence, but the Court will balance the risk of harm against the precautionary measures taken to avoid it in terms of time, trouble or money. So if a patient with known suicidal tendencies throws himself out of a window the Court will want to know what precautions were taken to avoid his doing that. It is worth remembering that shortage of staff is not an excuse that will be accepted because if, as a professional person, you realize that staffing is at a dangerous level then the onus is on you to try to rectify the situation, or at least to consider what action ought to be taken to avoid any ill effects to the patient.

Similarly, with violent patients who are also unpredictable and likely to injure themselves or others, a nurse must be able to show that she has at least given the situation some thought and has taken any necessary steps to avoid damage. Should a patient need to be restrained then great care must be taken to make sure that he comes to no harm. Where a patient is restrained unnecessarily he will have a case against the nurse for *false imprisonment* (which is another tort). If visitors are aggressive and threatening they should be removed by security officers. Where patients have known allergic responses or have previously reacted badly to drugs, a nurse must be able to show that she had considered the possibility and was prepared for the consequences, e.g. that the resuscitation tray was within easy reach.

The other groups of people who are particularly vulnerable are young children, mental defectives, and confused people. They cannot be held responsible for their own actions and consequently greater care is needed to ensure that their stay in hospital is free of legal difficulties.

Where there is an action for negligence a nurse may be able to show that the damage resulted from the actions of a third person and could not be directly linked to her. However, there are cases where such an act may be reasonably foreseeable, as with children, and in these cases there is no break in the chain of causation.

Also, if a patient consents to a course of treatment and subsequently suffers damage he will have no claim in negligence provided that the consent he gave was an informed consent. He must have had the risks explained to him and the person obtaining the consent must make sure that he has understood the possible consequences. The patient should be given time to think about it and should never be asked for his consent while under the influence of premedication or drugs which might impair his ability to think clearly. Failure to get a consent could result not only in the nurse facing a charge of negligence but also of assault and battery. However, should a patient arrive in a casualty department unconscious and in desperate need of medical attention, it would be negligent in those circumstances not to treat him. Where children are involved and the parents refuse to consent to treatment, then that child can be made a Ward of Court and the Court will grant consent if it is in the child's best interest to do so. Generally, obtaining the consent to an operation is the doctor's duty.

Nurses should beware of the pitfall of giving drugs on verbal prescriptions as such a practice is unsafe and probably illegal. Where a prescription sheet is illegible the nurse should make sure that it is rewritten, especially as drugs with very similar names have very different actions. If the prescribed dose is not that which is usually given, this discrepancy should be questioned before the drug is given to the patient, as a failure to do so would be negligence on the nurse's part.

Provided a nurse does not step outside her role and takes care over her work she should never find herself the subject of litigation. Generally the Court will only hold her responsible for the consequences of those wrongful acts which were reasonably foreseeable. The period of limitation for negligence is three years from the date that the patient realized that something was wrong. With children this time will continue to run from the date of their 18th birthday. This could mean that a child damaged *in utero* could sue any time up to his 21st birthday.

Where a patient's property is given into the care of nursing staff the belongings should be carefully and simply recorded. Precious metals should be described as such only if the nurse has taken the trouble to look for the hallmark. Money should be counted and recorded and preferably the entry should be countersigned. Where property is given into the care of hospital staff the hospital authority is liable for any loss, damage to or difference in description of those belongings. There is seldom a need to burn or destroy property and where this happens the hospital is obliged to replace it. If the patient insists on looking after his own items then any loss or damage is his responsibility.

Another tort which may concern the nurse is that of defamation – slander in its verbal form, libel where it is written or otherwise recorded. To prove defamation a patient would have to prove that what was said or written had lowered his good name in the eyes of right-thinking people, that it had referred to him and was published (i.e. made known), that it was prompted by malice, and that it was untrue. An action for defamation is unlikely in hospital. A more likely occurrence is a breach of confidence on the nurse's part, which, whilst it is unethical, is not actionable. Should a nurse's records be read out in Court, the nurse need not worry about being sued for defamation as she will be protected by privilege. Should outsiders such as the police wish to have access to patients' notes, they should seek permission to examine them from the Hospital Administrator. Where patients' notes are needed as evidence in Court, the hospital can be compelled to produce them under the Civil Evidence Act 1968.

A nurse must be careful of what is written in records: they should be clearly written and as objective as possible. If a mistake is made in recording an event, that mistake should be crossed out and the correction written alongside it. Where necessary the correction should be dated and initialled. Tippex should not be used to remove mistakes, nor should strips of paper be glued over the error, as these can later be removed, revealing the original mistake. If records look as if they have been interfered with or are sloppily written, the Court may come to its own conclusions that might not be to the nurse's benefit. Nursing records are the property of the hospital (not the patient) and should only be shown to people authorized to see them and who are involved in the treatment of that patient. Likewise, information gleaned about the patient is confidential and should not be divulged without the patient's consent.

Anyone who holds himself out to have a particular skill is obliged to exercise it. Thus a nurse must exercise her skills at the level appropriate to that individual, from CNO down to student nurse. Any task may be delegated provided it is within the competence of that person to carry it out. Where a task has been properly delegated then the responsibility falls on the person who accepts it. Student nurses will be liable for their own mistakes but the question of delegation would be viewed more critically in their cases.

Where a patient is unsure whom to sue or where the

person involved is impecunious, then he can sue the health authority because of its vicarious liability. Should the health authority have a large sum of money awarded against it, it is entitled to try to recover that money from its employee. Hence the necessity to join a professional body which will indemnify you up to a fixed amount against such an eventuality.

In conclusion, whilst law may seem an intimidating topic, when looked at from a practical point of view it is worth remembering that it has a positive side. It is protective and very few nurses have to face its punitive aspects. All a chapter like this can do is to increase your awareness of the legal implications of nursing and, having done that, prompt you to think before committing yourself to doing something which is outside your scope and capabilities. If you can answer 'yes' to the questions 'Can I justify my reasons for doing this?' and 'Can I stand on my own two feet?' then more than likely your nursing career will be free of legal complications.

Further reading

Hargreaves, M. (1979) *Practical Law for Nurses*. Pitman Medical.
Speller, S.R. (1976) *Law Notes for Nurses*. RCN.
Young, A. P. (1981) *Legal Problems in Nursing Practice*. (Lippincott Nursing Series). Harper & Row.

7

Clinical Nursing Research and the Staff Nurse

Vivien Coates

Introduction

'Nursing should become a research based profession; a sense of the need for research should become part of the mental equipment of every practising nurse and midwife.' The above statement was taken from the Briggs Report of the Committee on Nursing in 1972 and stresses that a scientific foundation must be the basis of nursing practice.

The discipline of nursing research has developed considerably in the past 20 years. For example, funds have been made available for conducting research studies and also for publishing research reports. Nurse research posts such as that of Research Liaison Officers have been instigated to help promote the undertaking and the use of nursing research within health regions. In acknowledgement of this progress the then General Nursing Council in 1977 decided that research must be incorporated into the training of registered nurses under the heading of 'Research Appreciation'. In the same year the Joint Board of Clinical Nursing Studies as it was then known also became committed to furthering nursing research and published *'The Research Objectives in Joint Board Courses'* which stated the intention to promote the concept of research mindedness: the ability to read, evaluate, select and make use of relevant findings. However, the time and effort which has been put into nursing research so far is most evident in the academic field. It was noted by Maura Hunt (1981) that little research is as yet put into practice: 'There is as yet no evidence that research is having any impact on nursing practice or that practitioners perceive research as having any direct relevance for practice' (M. Hunt 1981).

What is nursing research?

Part of the problem when attempting to interest nurses in research is that it may seem to be an academic exercise with little relevance to nursing practice. However, if the meaning of the word 'research' is explained it may make the activity seem more acceptable.

The definition offered by the *Oxford Paperback Dictionary* states that research is a 'careful study and investigation, especially in order to discover new facts or information'. As described by Clarke and Hockey (1979), research is 'an attempt to increase available knowledge by the discovery of new facts through systematic scientific enquiry'. Or, even more simply as defined by Treece and Treece (1977) 'research in its broadest sense is an attempt to gain solutions to problems'.

Nursing research, therefore, need not be an unintelligible activity undertaken by academics but rather it is a thorough investigation of virtually any nursing problem that might occur. The information yielded by the study may then be of use to nurses dealing with the problem in practice.

In this chapter so far it has been noted that nursing authorities (such as the GNC or JBCNS, now the English National Board and the ENB Post Basic Clinical Studies Courses) accept that research must be an integral part of nursing practice, and also that research findings may shed light on problems encountered when giving practical nursing care. It must now be argued that the role of the Staff Nurse should also include a commitment to the incorporation of research into nursing practice. Many of the issues covered in this book so far relate to the immediate concerns of the newly qualified Staff Nurse. The initial preoccupation when first left to manage the ward does usually relate to practical concerns. Such tasks as ensuring that patients receive the right treatment and are correctly prepared for investigations, that relatives are suitably attended to, that paperwork is up to date and that staff are organized tend to be the newly qualified nurse's primary interest. However, as the nurse gains ability and confidence as a ward manager, the wider aspects of the role of Staff Nurse need to be considered.

In addition to the day-to-day organization of the ward the Staff Nurse has a responsibility to ensure that she delivers a high standard of nursing care to her patients. During training nurses are often on a ward only long enough to grasp the essentials of nursing patients with a particular condition. However, the Staff Nurse is on a ward for a greater length of time and therefore has the opportunity both to improve her skills and to consider the nursing care given to patients in greater depth. As she deals with many patients with similar conditions and works with individuals for a prolonged time, the Staff Nurse has a chance to question the effect of current practice and to consider if various alternative methods of nursing care have anything of value to offer. When considering her own standards of practice the nurse must, if her nursing is to be based on reason rather than intuition, be prepared to judge the relevance of the contribution that nursing research can make towards quality clinical practice.

Crow (1981) investigated the relationship between research and standards of nursing care and concluded that in certain conditions research could contribute to nursing standards. It is not suggested that the findings of any research study could (or should) be uncritically applied to clinical nursing. However, if the findings of a valid investigation are applied to the appropriate situation they may be able to improve the quality of care received by the patient.

Although research is a comparatively new discipline in nursing, nurses may be surprised by both the amount of research work that is available and the extent to which it relates to practical nursing care. Early research studies generally concentrated upon issues concerned with nurses (for example, the 'ideal' personality of the nurse), nursing history, administration or education and paid less attention to the activity of nurses. However, over the last 20 years the emphasis has changed towards investigations into the actual practice of nursing.

The situation which has now evolved is that relevant information that has the potential to improve standards of care is available but is not being put into practice on the ward. For example, several studies have demonstrated the beneficial effects of thoroughly informing patients about their treatment (Boore 1978, Hayward 1975, Wilson-Barnett 1978) and yet nurse/patient communication is often a very brief and superficial activity.

Recording a patient's temperature is one of the first procedures taught to nurses; it is often a basis for further treatment and yet research findings (Nichols and Kuchas 1972) have illustrated that the recommended procedure gives inaccurate results. Thompson (1981) investigated the recording of patients' blood pressure and nurses should be aware of his recommendations to help ensure correct results. The above are only a few of the many examples that could be given to illustrate that available research is often not used.

The Staff Nurse, clinical research and tuition

When considering the wider aspects of the Staff Nurse's role it is also acknowledged that she has a responsibility for the instruction of learners. She teaches both through practical example and verbal instruction (see chapter 3). However, in addition to basing her own nursing care on science, the Staff Nurse must also encourage learners to question the rationale behind their actions. Therefore when teaching others the Staff Nurse must be prepared to link her tuition to substantiated information rather than perpetuating reliance upon tradition.

As pointed out by Murphy (1971), tradition is frequently based upon 'the transmission of superstition, speculation and the accumulation of unrationalised experiences'. Care which is based upon long taught procedures may originate from the personal preference of one Ward Sister. For example, Norton et al. (1959) found that regular turning of patients could significantly reduce the incidence of pressure sores, whilst the use of skin applications such as zinc or antiseptic creams was unsatisfactory. However, nurses continue to 'spray' and 'cream' pressure areas and to turn patients less regularly than is needed, usually according to the dictates of ward routine practice.

Jennifer Hunt (1981) has suggested five reasons why practitioners do not make use of research information, as follows:

1 They do not know about them.
2 They do not understand them.
3 They do not believe in them.
4 They do not know how to apply them.
5 They are not allowed to use them.

Part of the problem obviously lies with nurse educators who must bring research reports to the attention of their learners and also teach them how to interpret them critically. For if nurses are interested in research from the onset of their career it is more likely that research will become an integral part of practice. As yet this is not occurring to an acceptable level. Bond (1981) noted that newly qualified Staff Nurses had often not had any guidance in their training and were unable to see its relevance in practice. If a nurse is to be able to implement nursing research information she must have the ability to decide if the results of a study are relevant to her area of practice. According to Myco (1980) this involves (a) knowledge of the study subject, and (b) technical knowledge of research methods and data analysis.

In a study undertaken by Myco (1980) she found that possible sources of information such as journals and libraries were not used by individual nurses on a regular basis, and that nurse educational programmes did not appear to contain a commitment to the inclusion of research information in their curricula.

In 1976 Lancaster recommended that at registration nurses should be able to undertake the following four objectives:

1 Read and interpret reports in their own fields of nursing so that they can keep up to date with current knowledge and,

where appropriate, base their own policy and practice on research findings.

2 Identify areas of nursing where research is needed and be aware of the boundaries of their own knowledge and of situations in which lack of information is a serious detriment to effective decision making.

3 Collaborate intelligently with researchers (nurses and others) whose work brings them into contact with nursing.

4 Discuss with patients any research in which they (the patients) are being asked to participate in the same way that they are called upon to discuss diagnostic measures prescribed to patients by medical staff.

Although few qualified nurses could at present undertake the four listed objectives they are realistic goals towards which nurses could aim to gain proficiency. It is vital that the qualified nurse is research minded if nursing is to become a research-based profession, and it is a quality which is well within the grasp of all nurses. As stated by Clarke and Hockey (1979), 'research mindedness is an attitude of mind rather than a specific skill or ability'. Staff Nurses are therefore urged to look at their own work critically and objectively. They should be able to search for reasons underlying accepted practice and be prepared to change if evidence shows this to be an advantage.

If research in nursing has been only briefly discussed during training it must become the concern of the nurse to make herself aware of the literature relevant to her area of practice. This may be done via the nursing press. Some journals (such as the *Journal of Advanced Nursing)* are concerned primarily with research studies; however the 'popular press', such as the *Nursing Times* or *Nursing Mirror* now publish more research-based articles. The School of Nursing staff, both tutors and librarians, should be able to offer advice to nurses wishing to increase their knowledge and understanding of nursing research. Many of the courses for qualified nurses now have a specified research content (for example, the ENB Post Basic Clinical Studies Courses mentioned earlier). Some hospitals have tutors available for the further education of qualified staff who may be able to help nurses wishing to gain research information. A few hospitals employ a nurse or resource person specifically to promote the understanding and use of nursing research amongst nursing staff, who would be able to offer practical advice to those wishing to undertake their own research project. Study days may also be of value. There are also groups such as the local research interest group whose members meet to discuss and inform each other about nursing research.

For any nurse whose interest develops to the extent that she would like to undertake a research project, she will need supervision and advice. Such help may be available from hospital tutors or perhaps medical staff, depending upon the intended area of investigation. Alternatively, university or polytechnic lectures, resource personnel such as the Regional Liaison Officer, or the Research Society of the Royal College of Nursing may be able to provide additional advice.

Conclusion and further reading

To conclude this chapter there are several references listed below which may be of help to people who wish to increase their knowledge of research, or who perhaps are interested in starting a project of their own. They are (with one exception) articles from journals, and should all be readily obtainable. If the title is not self explanatory a brief description of the article is also included.

Clarke J.M. and Hockey L. (1979) *Research for Nursing. A Guide for the Enquiring Nurse.* Aylesbury: HM&M. Provides an introduction to the research process and also briefly describes completed research projects mentioning both methods used and results. The practical application of the findings is also stressed.

Gott, M. (1979) Nursing research; how to plan and implement a project. *Nursing Times* 28 June, pp. 1089–1092.

Hunt, J. (1984) Step by step. *Nursing Mirror* 4 Jan, pp. 29–30. The research process is a framework upon which research projects are based to help ensure a sound study. The article explains the steps which comprise the process and how they work in practice.

Hunt, J. (1984) Bridging the gap. *Nursing Mirror* 21 March p. 32. Discusses four informal ways that may easily be adopted by nurses to ensure that research is correctly applied.

Hunt, M. and Hicks, J. (1983) Promoting research awareness in post basic nursing courses. *Nursing Times* 30 March, pp. 41–42.

Molyneux, R.A. (1984) Practical research by student nurses. *Nursing Times* 22 February, pp. 59–61. An introduction to the use of the structured interview technique. It describes a pilot study conducted by third-year nursing studies. The results of a study about communication in patient care concerning patients who have undergone diagnostic procedures are also included.

Smith, S. (1984) A beginner's guide to research. *Nursing Times* 30 May, pp. 64–67.

For nurses who are interested in gaining further research information about particular topics, perhaps related to their own area of practice, but do not know where to start looking, the *Nursing Research Abstracts* are a helpful tool. These abstracts, which are an information service dealing with United Kingdom nursing research, are available in most academic libraries, and the librarian would be able to explain how to use them. The article listed below may also be found to be of value as it explains more fully the purpose of these abstracts.

Stodulski, A.H. and Stafford, S.M. (1982) Disseminating nursing research information in the U.K; Nursing Research Abstracts from the Index of Nursing Research. *International Journal of Nursing Studies* Vol. 19, No. 4, pp. 231–236.

References

Bond, S. (1981) *Research: a Base for the Future.* University of Edinburgh Nursing Studies Research Unit, pp. 31–40.

Boore, J. (1978) *A Prescription of Recovery.* RCN.

Department of Health and Social Security (1972) Report of the Committee on Nursing (Briggs Report). HMSO.

Clarke, J.M. and Hockey, L. (1979) *Research for Nursing. A Guide for the Enquiring Nurse.* HM&M.

Crow, R.A. (1981) Research and the standards of nursing care. *Journal of Advanced Nursing* Vol. 6 (No. 6), pp. 491–496.

General Nursing Council for England and Wales (1977) *Amended General Nursing Syllabus for the Register of Nurses.*

Hayward, J. (1975) *Information – a Prescription against Pain.* RCN.

Hunt, J. (1981) Indicators for nursing practice; the use of research findings. *Journal of Advanced Nursing* Vol. 6 (No. 3), pp. 189–194.

Hunt, M.W. (1981) Pathways to research in nursing practice. In: *Research: A Base for the Future.* University of Edinburgh Nursing Studies Research Unit, pp. 22–30.

Joint Board of Clinical Nursing Studies (1977) *The Research Objectives in Joint Board Courses.*

Lancaster, A. (1976) Towards a research based profession – 1. *Nursing Times* 22 April, pp. 632–633.

Murphy (1971) *Theoretical Issues in Professional Nursing.* Appleton Century Crofts.

Myco, J. (1980) Nursing research information: are nurse educators and practitioners seeking it out? *Journal of Advanced Nursing* Vol. 5 (No. 6), pp. 637–646.

Nichols, G.A. and Kuchas, D.H. (1972) Taking adult temperatures. Oral measurements. *American Journal of Nursing* Vol. 72, pp. 1091–1092.

Norton, D., McLaren, R. and Exton Smith, A.N. (1959) *An Investigation of Geriatric Nursing Problems.* Churchill Livingstone (1975 Reprint).

The Oxford Paperback Dictionary (1979) Oxford University Press.

Thompson, D.R. (1981) Recording patients' blood pressure; a review. *Journal of Advanced Nursing* Vol. 6 (No. 4), pp. 283–290.

Treece, E.W. and Treece, J.W. (1977) *Elements of Research in Nursing.* C.V. Mosby.

Wilson-Barnet, J. (1978) Patients' emotional responses to barium X-rays. *Journal of Advanced Nursing* Vol. 3 (No. 1), pp. 37–46.

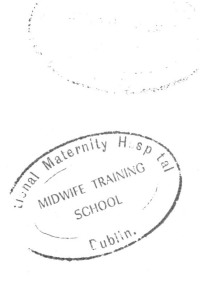

Information Technology and the Staff Nurse

S. Old

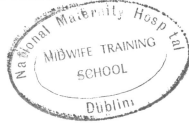

Introduction

The previous chapters have demonstrated that the newly qualified Staff Nurse has much to learn. There are many skills to develop and responsibilities to cope with. One such responsibility is to make use of any available resources in such a way that the patient may derive the most benefit.

Information technology is becoming an increasingly important resource within the National Health Service. Many nurses would rather ignore this resource but they do so at the risk of being negligent towards their patients. The NHS is facing a revolution of technology which nursing has to absorb and not ignore. If nurses do not involve themselves in the development and utilization of computer systems then the patients will most certainly suffer. Computers are all around us. We regularly use computer-based machines in our every day life; we even wear them on our wrists. There is an ever increasing use of computers in our education system. They can be found in primary, middle and secondary schools and in Schools of Nursing. I would therefore suggest that the newly qualified Staff Nurse is likely to know as much, if not a great deal more, about computers than her more senior colleagues. Many young nurses will consequently find themselves relied upon to play a significant role in assisting the ward team to adapt to new technology as it is introduced to the ward environment.

Information

If the term 'information technology' is considered, it becomes clear that computers are in the business of handling information. Anyone working within the NHS will be well aware of the importance that is attached to effective communication and record keeping. This has been recently demonstrated by the establishment of the Steering Group on Health Service Information set up in 1980 under the chairmanship of Mrs Edith Körner. This group was set up to look specifically at the masses of data that flow between all levels of the NHS. There are significant implications for the use of information technology arising from the Körner group reports (Körner 1984). Computers are being seen as the only means of storing and collating the immense quantity of information that seems to be required in order to run the NHS effectively. Nurses are being faced with having to collect and communicate ever-increasing amounts of information. It has been suggested (Pritchard 1982) that many nurses feel that forms are regarded by some as more important than the patients. The same author, however, commented that the information recorded on such forms was often vital to the care of the patients. Errors in the prescribing and provision of care will most certainly occur if there is not effective communication between health care professionals.

The computer can be an invaluable tool for storing large amounts of information both safely and in such a form that it is readily available. It would thus appear that information technology could be a great asset to the nurse. Computers could relieve nurses of many administrative duties so that they could concentrate much more of their time on using their nursing skills to the benefit of the patients under their care.

How computers work

I have suggested that nurses need to involve themselves in the development and utilization of computer systems. I do not believe, however, that it is either desirable or necessary for nurses to become expert programmers or systems analysts. Nurses need only to understand enough about what computers have got to offer in order to explain nursing needs realistically to the computer specialists. It is important to remember that computers are electronic machines. They are most certainly complicated machines and consequently subject to misunderstanding and misuse but they have no intellect of their own.

Data entry

It was not long ago that most computers obtained their data via punched cards. Such cards were coded and entered into the computer in batches. The large main frame computers which are usually found at Regional centres often use a batch-loading technique but the user now fills in pre-printed forms with a pen rather than using punched cards. It is most usual to see data being entered into a computer via terminals consisting of a visual display unit (VDU) and a typewriter-style keyboard. Most of these keyboards incorporate 'function keys'. Each of these keys can perform a pre-set task which enables the user to enter data more quickly.

Techniques to assist the non-expert user in entering data into a computer are continually being developed. The light pen is one such development and enables you to select information from a screen display by simply placing the pen over the appropriate part of the screen. For the nurse who is not a typist this kind of development can make the difference between a useful computer system and one that is a hindrance. Considerable effort is at present being directed at producing a cost-effective device which will enable us to talk directly to computers. In the intensive care type environment it is possible to transfer data directly from monitors to computers. This has a direct effect on the workload of those nurses usually expected to manually record monitored information.

Data storage

The storage capacity (memory) of a computer is one of its most obvious attributes. Large amounts of data can be stored within the minute electrical circuits of a computer and with the assistance of magnetic tapes and discs whole libraries of information can be stored in a very small space. Computers are particularly good at performing repetitive tasks, as they are capable of storing groups of instructions (programs) as well as the data on which these instructions act.

Data manipulation

Computer programs can be considered to be of two types: sorting programs or mathematical programs. When performing sorting tasks the computer is acting as an automatic filing cabinet. Data once entered into the system can be duplicated and stored in any number of files. The sorting process is also able to arrange the data in each file so that easily understood records are produced. This type of process is of considerable value when we consider the multi-professional nature of the NHS. All groups of health professionals require information about patients if they are to fulfil their role in the care of these patients. A certain amount of information about a patient will be required by one professional group only, but a great deal of information is relevant to more than one group. By using a computer system, data need only be collected once, and each professional group can be provided with the information it requires – arranged in a format which complements its mode of practice.

Computers are capable of performing lengthy calculations on large amounts of data at great speed. Nurses are required to perform many calculations in the course of their duties. Drug dilutions have to be calculated and checked, dietary intakes assessed and, in her role as a ward manager, the nurse has a considerable amount of work involving the collation of figures. This work is necessary if the patient is to be safely cared for, but it does take up a lot of time. If the computer can perform many of these tasks automatically, then both the nurse and patient will derive considerable benefit.

Data retrieval

Probably one of a computer system's most valuable attributes is its ability to transfer information from one place to another at great speed. There are various forms that the retrieval of information can take. Information can be displayed on VDUs for casual referral, or it can be printed out for manual filing in the more traditional manner.

Summary

Computers are complicated electronic machines capable of storing large amounts of data. This data can be manipulated, duplicated or analysed and information can be presented in the required form at the appropriate time and place.

Where are computers in nursing?

The introduction of information technology in the NHS has been widespread. Some of the systems currently in use are summarized in Table 1. The summary is far from definitive but it does demonstrate just how far-reaching the influence of computers in health care has been. There can be few areas of activity within either the hospital or community environments that have not been subject to the introduction of computer technology.

Most computer systems in use within the NHS have had some effect on nurses, but there are three types of system to which the nurse should pay particular attention. Firstly there are those systems that have been designed exclusively to assist the nurse in the performance of her duties, e.g. nursing record systems. There are then those systems which are involved in particular areas of activity which concern patient care but involve other groups of staff as well as nurses, e.g.

Chapter 8

Table 1 Computer systems in health care

Area of use	Applications
Clinical	Clinical nursing records
	Care plans
	Nursing procedures
	Drug information
	Patient monitoring
	Closed-loop therapy
	Computer-aided diagnosis
Management	Nurse/patient dependency
	Nurse allocation
	Personnel records
	Sickness/absence records
Education	Nurse training records
	Computer-assisted learning
	Computer manager learning
Primary/Community care	Child health registers
	Patient records
	Immunization records
Administrative	Master patient index
	In-patient records
	Waiting lists
	Out-patient appointments
	Scheduling of operating lists
	Payroll
	Manpower planning
	Accounting
Departmental	Laboratory systems
	Stock control
	Pharmacy
	Diagnostic imaging
	X-ray
Research	Data storage
	Statistical analysis

drug prescription and administration systems. Finally there are the systems which deal with large-scale organizational matters that affect the management of the patients that nurses care for, e.g. patient administration systems. The value of these systems can be demonstrated by considering their applications.

Nursing care and the computer

Many hospitals and companies have developed computer-based nursing record systems. Three hospitals have been particularly successful in developing such systems: The Royal Devon and Exeter Hospital, Wonford, The Queen Elizabeth Hospital, Birmingham, and Ninewells Hospital, Dundee. When considering the value of a computer system to nurses it is worth remembering that the primary role of a nurse is to provide care for her patients. Any computerized nursing record system must thus ensure that the nurse is enabled to spend more time with the patients under her care. Nurses have to spend a considerable proportion of their time recording all they want to do and all they have done. Nurses are also expected to act as recording clerks for other health professionals. As the administrative workload of the nurse increases, the amount of time a nurse spends in direct contact with the patient decreases. This problem cannot be solved by simply recording less information. For an individual patient to receive planned and consistently good care from a constantly changing team of nurses it is necessary to accurately record and communicate a mass of information.

Computers are being used as a tool to assist nurses in the systematic organization of the delivery of care to the patient. Screen displays have been designed to assist the nurse to record care activities. Activities of daily living, diagnostic categories and activities associated with physiological systems are all frameworks around which this type of screen display has been designed. To save time, care activities are usually selected from 'menus' displayed on the screen by using a light pen or a single key on the keyboard. Some

95

systems use lists of commonly used phrases so that coherent nursing orders can be constructed with ease.

All nursing record systems need to be designed with the nurse in mind. Consequently you will find that in order to operate the best computerized nursing record system, very little longhand typing is required. The importance of ward-based nursing staff contributing to the design of the computerized nursing system cannot be overemphasized. The amount of planning that goes into the production of a system will determine how effective it is. If commonly used activities are not included in the menu displays of a system then the nurse will find herself taking more time to record care on the computer system than if she had used a manual system.

Care planning

There is often so much to write in a care plan and the patient's required care changes so rapidly that nurses avoid writing them. Computerized systems can make the initial writing of care plans easier by providing standard formats to follow. Updating is also easier as care plans can be recalled and amended via a computer terminal.

Computer systems can also assist in the scheduling of care; the Sister or Staff Nurse in charge of the ward can be provided with workload summaries. If it is appropriate that certain orders should only be operational for a set length of time then these can be automatically erased by the system, as required.

To assist in the delivery of care, computer systems can store instruction lists. Whenever a nursing order involving tests or investigations is displayed, the appropriate instruction list can be automatically displayed with the order.

Recording care

Care can be recorded either via the computer terminal or by signing a computer print-out that can then be stored in standard files.

To allow for continuity of care it is normal for a system to provide a cumulative history of nursing care. This enables easy evaluation of care and can be used after a patient's discharge as part of the nursing record. The writing of information in the standard Kardex can be considerably reduced, if not totally eliminated.

Evaluations of the effects of computerization on the nursing records (Kumpel and Davis 1982) have produced interesting results. Care plans have been found to be more accurate and complete. They are certainly more legible and easy to follow, due to better structuring. The use of often misunderstood abbreviations disappears and a more complete record of the care given to a patient is usually produced. Claire Ashton (1983b) states: 'There is no doubt that with improvement in the quality, quantity and availability of individualized patient information, communication, co-ordination, continuity and monitoring of care have been enhanced.'

Drug prescribing and administration

A computer system for the prescribing, dispensing and administration of drugs has been implemented at Queen Elizabeth Hospital, Birmingham. The system developed from a project established in 1969 as part of the experimental programme sponsored by the Department of Health and Social Security (DHSS). The stated objectives of this system were:

1 To improve the quality of prescribing by ensuring that at the time of prescribing the doctor has as much information as possible about the patient and the proposed drug treatment.

2 To prevent the prescribing of inappropriate or potentially dangerous drugs by the use of checking procedures.

3 To reduce errors in drug administration by the provision of a printed administration document with clear, unambiguous prescriptions.

4 To provide a data base for studies of prescribing patterns and for detecting and monitoring adverse drug reactions.

Prescribing

A doctor wishing to prescribe a drug for a patient first has to 'log' into the system using a personal code. Every doctor has a unique code and thus it is possible for the system to identify who has prescribed each drug. The doctor uses a standard keyboard and VDU for entering and recalling information from the system. Most entries can be made by selecting items from menus or by filling in questionnaire type forms displayed on the screen. In order for the computer system to attain information about a patient the doctor has to fill in a questionnaire before the first drug is prescribed.

Once the doctor has selected the patient and the drug he wishes to prescribe he is automatically presented with a display of information concerning the suitability of the drug for that patient. This display includes a summary of the patient's current prescriptions and associated information concerning contraindications and hypersensitivities. The computer checks the selected drug against the patient's age, questionnaire information, his current prescription and the most recent laboratory data.

The computer system does not prevent the doctor from prescribing any drug that he wishes but if contraindication warnings are ignored, then a print-out of the prescription is automatically produced in the pharmacy department.

The doctor can select the route, frequency and dosage of a drug from a standard display or he can use a free text facility, if the prescription is of an irregular nature.

When the doctor has completed a prescription it is displayed for confirmation. Once confirmed a prescription list is printed on a ward printer. The prescription list is similar in design to a standard prescription chart. All of the usual details are included: name, age, unit no., date and time of the drug due, etc.

Drug administration

The nurse's responsibilities when administering medication to a patient are no different when using a computer system than a manual system. The nurse is still required to ensure that the right patient receives the correct drug at the appropriate time. The drug administration chart also requires the usual nurse signature after each drug has been administered.

Drug dispensing

In addition to information concerning contraindicated drug prescriptions, the hospital pharmacy also uses the computer system for stock control. If a drug is prescribed on a ward which does not usually stock that drug then the pharmacy is automatically informed that the drug requires dispensing. The system also deals with the dispensing of the drugs which the patient requires to take out when discharged (TTOs).

System benefits

The doctor and nurse, and consequently the patient, can derive considerable benefit from this system. It offers both added safety and saved time.

Safety Nurses have no difficulty reading the printed prescription and as incomplete prescriptions will not be accepted by the computer, errors in the administration of drugs are less likely to occur. Doctors are less likely to make prescribing errors as they are provided with a complete set of relevant information concerning the suitability of each drug they prescribe for their patients. The patient is thus more likely to receive appropriate medication and, because prescription charts never have to leave the ward in order for drugs to be dispensed, the patient is more likely to receive new medication at the earliest possible time.

Time In a labour-intensive organization like the NHS, time is money. If Figure 1 is considered, it can be seen that the system can save the doctor and nurse time because it automatically transfers information from one area to another. The computer system is thus creating closed information loops. For example, the computer can receive biochemistry results

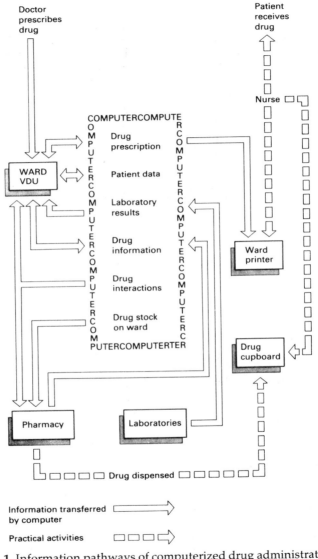

Fig. 1 Information pathways of computerized drug administration system.

as soon as they are available – directly from the laboratory. These results are then automatically filed in the appropriate records. The nurse consequently does not have to spend time transcribing telephone messages or searching for lost results slips. The pharmacy link will offer similar advantages. Stock control is automatic. The nurse will spend less time searching for drugs which are not in stock and will find it easier to find the drugs she requires because ward stocks are likely to be more regularly reviewed by the pharmacy.

This type of system has a lot to offer the whole ward team. Nurses must not underestimate the value of any drug system which enables the patient to receive any aspect of his treatment both safely and efficiently. If we consider that the course of a patient's treatment in hospital is often dependent on the speed with which test results can be obtained and therapy commenced, then we may find that this type of computer system actually reduces the patient's length of stay in hospital.

Intensive care

Before leaving the subject of patient care it is worth considering the use of computers in the intensive care environment. Technology has always been associated with specialist units, caring for the critically ill, and computers were first introduced to these units over 20 years ago. As surgical techniques and medical science have progressed, the requirement for monitoring various patient parameters has increased. The nurse working in the high dependency areas has had to cope with the resulting increase in technological equipment. The demand on the nursing time required to record monitored parameters is colossal.

Computer technology was originally seen by many nurses as just another barrier between themselves and the patient. Many nurses have now realized that computer systems can considerably reduce the record keeping duties of the nurse. Systems have been used to gather data automatically from different monitors and to provide graphical or digital displays which assist the doctors and nurses in assessing a patient's condition. Alarm and clinical status prediction systems have been developed (Crew et al. 1984) in the cardiothoracic intensive therapy unit at Killingbeck Hospital, Leeds, as part of a DHSS-funded research project.

Although these systems have undergone only limited trials they potentially offer the nurse considerable support in the detection of the life-threatening events that inevitably occur in the care of the critically ill patient. The use of computer technology in high dependency areas is increasing rapidly along with the trend towards the automation of many activities, e.g. closed loop therapy. The nurse working in this environment has to consider very carefully how she should make use of the technology that surrounds her. Computers are only valuable tools if used as tools, and the nurse must guard against nursing computers rather than the patients.

Patient administration

Although a computerized Patient Administration System (PAS) would appear to have little to do with the staff nurse, it is likely to be the first system with which she has contact. Some of the systems have ward-based VDU facilities but the nurse is usually involved in filling in forms used to enter bed state data into the system. It is unfortunate that often the nurse is totally unaware of how this data is used.

A PAS contains a master index which consists of information about every patient entering the hospital. This information includes the patient's name, age, sex, address and General Practitioner. Patients are included in the master index whether they have attended the hospital as an in-patient or merely for an out-patient appointment. A history of a patient's admissions, discharges and out-patient appointments is built up within the system. A PAS is usually capable of formulating waiting lists and scheduling out-patient appointments. The system is also used to produce bed occupancy figures, real-time bed states and hospital activity statistics. The implications of the Körner group reports (Körner 1984) mean that District Health Authorities will be standardizing the format of hospital activity data produced by the Patient Administration Systems. This will enable managers to evaluate more effectively the facilities provided both within and between District Health Authorities.

Patient benefits

The patient can derive considerable benefit from a well organized PAS. The system can predict bed occupancy more accurately and consequently a higher bed occupancy and less cancellations of list admissions can result. The waiting list patient is therefore likely to receive hospital care more quickly and is less likely to suffer the psychological trauma of numerous alterations to his admission date.

The nurse's role

The nurse is responsible for collecting information about a patient's stay in hospital. Details of a patient's Consultant and diagnosis as well as transfer and discharge information are usually entered into the PAS by the ward nurse. In return the system does not offer the nurse much more than an efficient service in terms of the supply of patient data and medical records. However, the future development of hospital computer networks, based around administration systems, is likely to be of significant value to both nurse and patient.

Networks

Patient Administration Systems can form the hub around which most hospital computer systems could revolve (Figure 2).

Whether we consider a drug prescription system, a laboratory system or a nursing record system, the information contained in the master index element of a PAS is required by all of them. At present it is common to find a nurse transcribing patients' details from one form to another. Laboratory specimens, drug charts and care plans all need to be identified with the correct patient. Despite the availability of

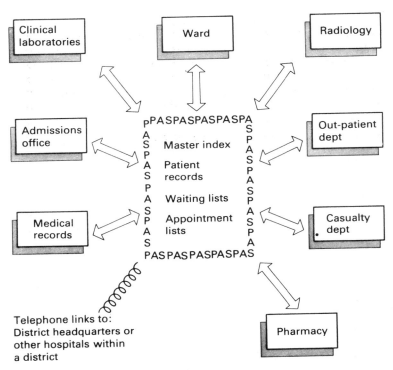

Fig. 2 The possible scope of a hospital computer network.

patient data stickers it would be much more efficient if a patient's details were automatically available to each department via a computer system.

This approach would also make the introduction of computer technology more cost effective. It is much easier to justify the expenditure required to supply every ward with a VDU when several systems are linked together. The time spent by the ward nurse entering information into this kind of computer network would be insignificant compared to the amount of time that could be saved by the system – relieving the nurse from many administrative and record-keeping duties. The computer system, for example, could deal with a patient's meal orders, dispensing drugs to the ward, the requisition of stores and scheduling patients' investigations. The possibilities seem to be limited only by our imagination.

The kind of computer links that can be achieved have significant implications for nurse managers. For example, patient dependency information could be extracted from a nursing record system and correlated with bed occupancy statistics from a PAS. The nurse manager would then have available the necessary information to identify the facilities and manpower required to provide an adequate service to the patient.

Nurse education

The Staff Nurse must never forget that she has both a responsibility concerning the education of students and a responsibility to ensure that her own educational development is maintained. Computer-assisted learning (CAL) is playing an increasingly important role in the education of many students and there is no reason why this technique could not be used in the ward environment.

There are several ways in which computers can assist the learner. They can for example be used to guide the learner through tutorials or to test her understanding of various concepts. Nurse tutors have also used computers to simulate clinical situations or body systems. One advantage of CAL is that the learner can work through problems at her own pace. The tutor can also be more flexible and concentrate on using her skills to cater more adequately for the individual needs of the learners.

Computer-assisted learning could therefore be an invaluable tool for improving the scope and quality of our education service.

Confidentiality

Confidentiality is a subject that nurses cannot ignore when considering the computerization of the patient's record. As a society we are becoming more and more concerned with the potential threats to an individual's privacy.

Nurses are responsible for safeguarding the personal information that they receive in the course of their duties. The nursing record of a patient is often likely to contain some information imparted confidentially by the patient or patient's relatives. If we intend to computerize the nursing record then we must ensure that the access to sensitive information is restricted.

It has to be said that many computer systems offer more security than their manual counterparts. However, this should not lead us into becoming complacent about the issue. There will always need to be a compromise between the ease of use of a system and its security. The nurse has the responsibility to represent the patient's interests and ensure that adequate security is maintained.

Table 2 The Younger Committee's Principles (Para 592–599)

---

1 Information should be regarded as held for a specific purpose and not be used without appropriate authorization for other purposes.

2 Access to information should be confined to those authorized to have it for the purpose for which it was supplied.

3 The amount of information collected should be the minimum necessary for the achievement of a specified purpose.

4 In computerized systems handling information for statistical purposes, adequate provision should be made in their design and programs for separating identities from the rest of the data.

5 There should be arrangements whereby the subject could be told about the information held concerning them.

6 The level of security to be achieved by a system should be specified in advance by the user and should include precautions against the deliberate abuse or misuse of information.

7 A monitoring system should be set up to facilitate the detection of any violation of the security of the system.

8 In the design of information systems periods should be specified beyond which information should not be retained.

9 Data held should be accurate, and there should be machinery for the correction of inaccuracy.

10 Care should be taken in coding value judgements.

A considerable amount of national activity has concerned itself with the confidentiality of records. Several Bills concerned with data protection have been passed through Parliament since the early 1960s. Mrs Körner's Steering Group on Health Service Information set up its own working group specifically to consider this issue. The legislation on data protection and confidentiality is likely to be amended frequently over the next decade as the ramifications of the developments in the field of information technology are fully realized. As far as nurses are concerned, the Younger Committee's principles, as summarized in Table 2, form a good guide to follow when considering computer systems and confidentiality (Younger 1972).

Good or bad systems

If the information needs of nursing are not fully considered when a computer system is being selected then an inadequate system will most certainly result. Computers are only machines and as such their capabilities are limited by the imagination and skill of the programmer.

Unfortunately, ward-based nursing staff are rarely consulted about the type of hospital computer system to be installed. However, they should not be silent when faced with systems which do not fulfil their expectations. Although it is most certainly costly, and often impossible to make major changes to an up and running computer system, small modifications can be made to make the system more acceptable to the user. Acceptable systems suitable to nursing needs will only develop if ward level staff are prepared to make a critical appraisal of the systems they use.

Three basic problems have been identified (Cook 1982) which can be either diminished or accentuated, depending on whether a good or bad computer system is developed: proliferating paperwork, increased volume and complexity of information, and escalating costs.

Proliferating paperwork

Estimates of the amount of time that nurses spend processing paperwork vary enormously (30% Cook 1983; 70% Berg 1983). However, it is only too evident that a large administrative work load is often placed upon the shoulders of even the most junior of Staff Nurses. The earlier descriptions of computer systems have demonstrated that a good system can relieve the nurse from many of these duties. On the other hand, if a system is not well designed it can make matters a great deal worse. A bad system may omit to take care of time-consuming details. Information may not be produced to the user's specification, leading to the tedious task of sifting through computer printouts to find a vital snippet of information. Excess or duplicated information can be produced by poorly specified systems, which again only serves to confuse the user, causing time and effort to be wasted.

Increased volume and complexity of information

A well designed computerized patient information system can organize the large volume of complex information that is required in order to care for patients adequately. Formats can be designed so that the user finds it easy to assess the information being presented, and check lists can be provided to assist in the collection of data. However, the problem of handling large amounts of complex information will be made considerably worse if information loops are not closed. A system that either requires the entry or retrieval of data using methods that are not compatible with the normal practice of the nurse will lead to the inaccurate recording of data, and consequently a poor quality of information.

Escalating costs

If a computer system can save a nurse time then the cost of care per patient can be reduced. Conversely, if a computer system is either difficult to operate or has to run alongside back-up manual systems due to its unreliability, then time and consequently money will be wasted.

What makes a good system?

To be really useful a computer system must perform either time-consuming or difficult tasks. The system certainly needs to be both easy to operate and reliable. Computer systems also need to be able to protect their data so that both sensitive information is kept secure and important information is not lost. A system is of real value when it improves the communication between medical, nursing and ancillary services, whilst reducing the manual requirement for information transfer.

Conclusion – the nurse's role

However good a computer system might be, users of the system will have to undergo some kind of training. Nurse managers and tutors have got to ensure that ward-based nursing staff are provided with the support and training required.

Nurses in general have got to evaluate how they can best utilize the technology that is offered to them. When considering the value of any particular system they have to ask themselves whether the system will help them provide better care for their patients. Nurses who ignore the words of Professor Kathryn Hannah (1978) do so at the risk of doing an injustice to themselves and their patients: 'The use of computers in client care will be the biggest change to confront nurses and nursing in the next decade. In the nursing profession we are just beginning to experience the profound impact that computers will ultimately have on nursing practice and patient care. No longer is the question 'Should our profession resist automation?' The question now becomes 'How do we cope with the resisting forces within and among ourselves so that the result is a stable, predictable, rational approach to improving the quality of nursing practice and thus the quality of patient care?'

There is immense potential for the use of computers in nursing to the benefit of both nurse and patient. The ward nurse, with the help of information technology, can ensure that her primary role remains that of caring for the patient. However this will only occur if nurses grasp the opportunities to involve themselves fully in the development of Health Service computer systems. The young computer-literate Staff Nurses of today have a great responsibility to guide their professional colleagues in the right direction. Nurses make up 48% of the workforce within the NHS and as such have a right to make their voices heard. We must free ourselves of any reluctance to involve ourselves in what we might think is a non-nursing matter. Nursing expertise is essential to ensure that the right balance is achieved between the humanitarian needs of the patient and the use of technology. Information technology can be made to work for us but the choice is ours, and ours only.

References

Ashton, C.C. (1983a) Caring for patients within a computer environment, pp. 105–114 in Scholes et al. (1984).

Ashton, C.C. (1983b) A computer system for drug prescribing and its impact on drug administration, pp. 174–196 in Scholes et al. (1984).

Berg, C.M. (1983) The importance of nurses' input for the selection of computerised systems, pp. 42–58 in Scholes et al. (1984).

Cook, M. (1982) Using computers to enhance professional practice. *Nursing Times* 15 September, pp. 1542–1544.

Cook, M. (1983) Using computers to enhance professional practice, pp. 84–90 in Scholes et al. (1984).

Crew, A.D., Stoodley, K.D.C., Naghdy, F. & Unsworth, G.D. (1984) Preliminary studies in the identification of cardiac status in a cardiac surgical intensive therapy unit. In: *Intensive Care Medicine*, pp. 71–79. Springer-Verlag.

Hannah, K.J. (1978) Computers and nursing. *Hospital Administration in Canada* Vol. 20 (No. 5), pp. 20–23.

Körner, E. (1984) The Steering Group on Health Service Information.

Third Report from Working Group E to the Secretary of State. DHSS.

Kumpel, Z. and Davies, A. (1982) Quantitative evaluation of the effects of computerisation on the nursing record. *Proceedings of MIE* Vol. 82, pp. 336–342.

Pritchard, K. (1982) Computers 3: possible applications in nursing. *Nursing Times* 17 March, pp. 465–466.

Scholes, M., Bryant, Y. and Barber, B. (eds) (1982) *The Impact of Computers in Nursing: An International Review.* Elsevier North-Holland.

Younger, K. (1972) *Report of the Committee on Privacy.* HMSO (Cmnd 5012).

Further reading

Bradbeer, R., De Bono, P. & Laurie, P. (1982) *The Computer Book.* BBC.

Frates, J. & Moldrop, W. (1980) *Introduction to the Computer, An Integrated Approach.* Prentice-Hall.

Hannah, K.J. & Ball, M.J. (eds) (1984) *Using Computers in Nursing.* Reston.

Jarrett, D. *The Good Computing Book for Beginners.* EEC.

Kostrewski, B. (ed.) (1984) *Current Perspectives in Health Care Computing.* Cambridge University Press.

Norman, S.E. & Townsend, I. (eds) (1982) *Computers in Nurse Education. A Focused Bibliography 1962–1982.* NHS Learning Resources Unit, Sheffield.

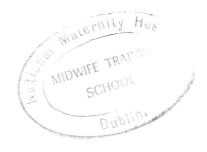

9

What Next?

Angela Senior

Introduction

'So You Passed, Nurse', the title of a nursing education research project (Bendall 1975), is by now nationally known and often quoted. It begs the question 'What next?' With a licence to practise the nurse gives notice of the professional service she has to offer and this puts the onus on her to practise as a professional, giving informed, up-to-date care and service throughout her working life.

Nursing – your profession

This is perhaps a good time to examine nursing to see whether it possesses all the ingredients which would make it a legitimate profession; and if it does not, to highlight a missing ingredient which the newly registered nurse could help to establish and maintain.

'Nursing is in the throes of seeking professional status. in order to do this nurses must meet the requirements of society with the demands of a profession, that is: autonomy, distinctive expertness and control over practice and education' (Simms 1977).

Many writers, including Chapman (1977) and Pyne (1981), have attempted to describe the attributes of a profession. However much these differ in detail, they all boil down to much the same thing. It would seem that society grants a profession a mandate to do a job and to perform specific tasks based on a specialized body of knowledge. Autonomy seems

113

to be a key component and with it responsibility for action and accountability to its clients and to society.

Nursing's ideal claim to a specialized body of knowledge would be that which it has built up through research. It is only relatively recently, in the 1970s, that the first spate of nursing research appeared as a result of the 12 Royal College of Nursing (Rcn) research projects. These provided factual information about nursing practice and provided some theoretical bases for improvement of nursing care. In addition Chapman agrees that nursing draws on the behavioural sciences to produce theories of care in much the same way tha doctors draw on the natural and biological sciences to produce theories of diagnosis and cure. A good example of nursing's use of the behavioural sciences is the high quality nursing care given to children in hospital as a result of psychological studies of the development of children and maternal deprivation.

Autonomy? It is convincingly argued that nursing can never achieve autonomy because it never truly escapes medical direction. If one defines nursing as Virginia Henderson does – 'The unique function of the nurse is to perform for the individual, sick or well, those activities which contribute to health or its recovery (or to peaceful death) which he would perform unaided had he the necessary strength or will to do so' – and if one applies the Nursing Process in performing these activities for the client, then it could be argued that nurses can act autonomously. The nurse, drawing on her knowledge of the behavioural and biological sciences, uses her senses to assess the client in order to identify where nursing intervention is needed. She then plans the nursing intervention, taking into account medical and paramedical prescriptions of cure, and using skilled techniques implements the plan. Finally, she evaluates those actions and effects attributed to her nursing intervention. This should be seen as an autonomous function which is complementary to medicine but certainly not subservient to it. Furthermore, the nurse must assume responsibility for her intervention and is accountable to the patient, her colleagues and to society.

By statute, nursing does have control over practice and the education of its basic learners. As yet, there seems to be no formal organized system of continuing nurse education, and no great awareness amongst practising nurses of the contribution they could make to the development of such a system.

In 1970 a non-statutory body, the Joint Board of Clinical Nursing Studies (now absorbed into the statutory English National Board for Nursing, Midwifery and Health Visiting), was set up to oversee and direct specialist clinical nursing courses at the post-basic level – adding to the distinctive expertness of the nurse. As recently as 1981, three publications relating to the continuing education and training of nurses in the United Kingdom have emerged. These are the National Staff Committee for Nurses & Midwives' *The Organisation and Provision of Continuing In-service Education and Training,* The Auld Commission *Report on Continuing Education for the Nursing Profession in Scotland* and the National Health Service Staff Training Centre's *Report on Seminar – Professional Development in Clinical Nursing: The 1980s.* The Scottish document in its preamble warns that nurses who once thought that training ended with a successful result at State Final Examination must now realize that in order to keep pace with technological advancement they have 'to learn and re-learn throughout their professional lives'.

So what next? A deliberate and well resourced dynamic continuing education programme is needed constantly to update nursing's body of knowledge, to direct personal and professional advancement and, above all, to ensure a consistently high standard of patient care.

Existing continuing education opportunities

The term 'continuing education' is open to debate and in nursing is still under discussion within the UK and other EEC countries. It is perhaps simplest to consider it as a blanket term used to describe any planned form of education or training undertaken after a basic qualification, aimed at developing and maintaining the professional status and competence of the nurse, ultimately to improve nursing care. What seems to be emerging in the UK is a broad two-way division into:

1 Post-basic education
2 Professional and personal development

Post-basic education

The underlying theme here is that for entry to any form of post-basic study a basic nursing qualification is a prerequisite. The basic qualification forms the core of a new area of clinical practice. Study is at a deeper level of knowledge and skill development and is aimed at producing expertness in the chosen specialty.

Specialist clinical nursing courses

Such nursing courses are offered by approved Schools of Nursing, Polytechnics and Universities under the aegis of the Continuing Education and Training Department of the National Boards (formerly JBCNS in England and Wales and CCNS in Scotland). These courses are now described as Post-Basic Clinical Nursing Studies Courses, of which there are some 90 different specialties, such as renal nursing for Registered General Nurses, nursing care of the mentally handicapped in the community for Registered Nurses of the Mentally Subnormal, nursing care of the mentally ill in the community for Registered Mental Nurses, and so on. An up-to-date list of available courses and approved Centres is published at regular intervals by the Continuing Education and Training Departments of the National Boards and is circulated to Schools of Nursing and Continuing Education Departments in all District Health Authorities.

Crucial to any continuing education is the firm belief that the newly registered nurse requires a period of consolidation into her new role. Picture the young and relatively inexperienced Staff Nurse having to face the responsibilities and range of tasks expected of a trained member of the nursing team. There is obviously a need for her to 'find her feet' before embarking on any further study. For this reason another requirement for entry to in-depth Post-Basic Clinical Nursing Studies Courses ('long' courses) is a minimum period of six months post-registration experience, not necessarily in the chosen specialty. The other type of Post-Basic Clinical Nursing Studies Course (the 'short' course) is essentially an up-dating course for experienced nurses already working in the specialty, where the requirement is a minimum of two years post-registration experience with substantial experience in the specialty. A Post-Basic Clinical Nursing Studies course of choice is much recommended nowadays in preference to the once automatic move, often for the motive of purely personal advancement, to other Statutory Courses such as Midwifery and Mental Nursing.

Other statutory post-basic courses

These include a shortened period of training to qualify registered nurses to work in other nursing disciplines, e.g. Mentally Ill; Mental Handicap; Paediatrics; Midwifery; District Nursing; Orthopaedics; Ophthalmics. All Post-Basic Clinical Nursing Studies Courses can be pursued either on a secondment basis, i.e. with conditional support from the nurse's employing authority, or on a contract basis, where the nurse is employed by the authority mounting the course on a fixed contract for the duration of the course.

Professional and personal development

This area of continuing education can conveniently be subdivided into

(i) orientation
(ii) in-service training
(iii) professional development
(iv) personal development

(i) Orientation

Orientation introduces newly qualified and newly appointed nurses to the philosophy and aims of an institution, giving information on policy, procedures, physical facilities and special services. It also focuses on role expectation, through discussion giving hints for smooth transition from learner to trained status or from one grade to the next. For obvious reasons, orientation courses are provided immediately upon appointment and when there is a change in grade or status.

(ii) In-service training

This subdivision of continuing education covers the learning experiences and opportunities provided on the job, hence 'in-service'. The training is relatively specific to the job and to the institution. It is aimed at assisting the nurse to function efficiently in all aspects of her specialty and in having full knowledge and understanding of the overall policies and regulations related to her work.

Training is often informal, ranging from just two persons discussing a topic or working together in a clinical area to large groups participating in seminars, workshops, etc. in the classroom.

In-service training may include clinical practice and related theory, professional matters, or ward/hospital/Health Service policy. It may be pro-active, anticipating imminent change, such as the intensive in-service training programme carried out prior to the recent change of insulin to the new U100; or it may be re-active, such as revision of infection control measures when there is a rise in the incidence of, for example, infected wounds in a surgical ward.

(iii) Professional development

Professional development involves planned and organized learning experiences which build upon the knowledge and skills of the nurse. In the ideal situation learning needs are identified mainly through staff appraisal and performance review. The education and training provided here generally matches the level of responsibility of the nurse and continues to develop her communication, clinical and management skills. Professional development programmes for newly qualified nurses are run in all districts, in a variety of formats ranging from one day workshops to one or two week courses. This area of continuing education has been the subject of much consideration and future developments in this area are outlined later on in this chapter.

Further professional development courses include:

Management The principles of management apply in all branches of nursing, from the management of patient care in clinical practice to the management of educational processes, to the overall management of the nursing services at district, regional and national levels. Management courses are organized by District and Regional Health Authorities, mostly in association with Colleges of Further Education and other National Health and private training institutions. They cover training for first line managers (Charge Nurse/Clinical Teacher grade), middle managers (Senior Nurses/Nurse Tutor grade), senior management (Directors of Nursing Services, Directors of Nurse Education) and specialist managers (personnel, manpower, planning officers).

The management courses at middle and senior levels are usually multidisciplinary, but in recent years role based training for Directors of Nursing Services (Mentally Ill/Mentally Handicapped) has been introduced. The programme is led professionally by having senior managers as facilitators. It is based on linking learning to the individual manager's work-related problems, thus helping the individual to understand her role and to manage more effectively.

Education Although all nurses have a significant teaching role as part of the professional service they give, many are needed to educate and train future nurses as the major function of their role. There are a variety of education courses available, all based in Colleges of Further Education and Higher Education and some Universities. They prepare nurses to teach either primarily at the clinical level (Clinical Teachers) or primarily at the theoretical and educational management level (Nurse Tutors).

(iv) Personal development

Running concurrently with professional development is the personal development of the newly registered nurse. As in all other forms of continuing education, this depends very much on the nurse's own motivation. Even before qualifying many nurses have a fair idea of what they hope to achieve during their professional lives and recognize that it is important to plan their professional future accurately. Fulfilling the plan provides not only personal achievement but also job satisfaction and informed patient care.

There are a number of higher education opportunities for nurses, including the London University Diploma in Nursing, First and Higher Degree Courses, and DHSS Research Studentships. An encouraging point about these opportunities for higher education is that many of the institutions concerned will take into consideration basic nursing qualifications as part of the entrance requirement. Degree courses may be undertaken on a full-time, part-time or combined full- and part-time basis. Most health authorities will give financial assistance and/or paid study leave if it can be shown that the course or study undertaken will benefit the organization and improve the nurse's performance at work. Local Education Authority grants may be available to those who decide to study on a full-time basis at University or Polytechnic.

Professional organizations Membership of a professional organization, such as the Royal College of Nursing, opens the door to a wide range of activities and learning opportunities which can only enhance the nurse's personal security and professional status.

Career opportunities

Apart from the general career development principles outlined in the previous section, there are a number of options available to the newly registered nurse. Of note are opportunities to work in the Armed Forces, Prison Nursing Service, on board ship, Voluntary Service Overseas, and in the EEC. All registered nurses who commenced training on or after 29 June 1979 are eligible for freedom of movement throughout the member states of the EEC. Those who completed training before that date need to apply to the appropriate board of the United Kingdom Central Council for clarification of their eligibility to work in an EEC country. Advertised regularly in the nursing press and other professional agencies are research studentships, scholarships, business grants, etc., offered to nurses by the Department of Health and Social Services, Regional Health Authorities, professional organizations, charitable trusts, The Kings Fund Centre, and commercial and private firms.

Up-to-date information and details of professional development and career opportunities, including useful addresses, can be obtained from the Nursing and Health Service Careers Centre, 121/123 Edgware Road, London W2 2HX.

The future

Professional development in clinical nursing

This proposed component of continuing education for nurses in the United Kingdom is probably the most exciting development to date. It stems from early deliberation in the 1970s concerning standards of nursing care and the provision of a satisfactory career in clinical nursing. In September 1981, the Department of Health and Social Security organized a residental seminar focusing on the needs of the newly registered nurse. The main objective was 'to identify recently registered nurses, with particular regard to their individual responsibility for the effective practice of nursing now and in the future'.

From this 1981 seminar two principles emerged which set the scene for what should happen next. First was that professional development should be a continuous educational process; and second that accreditation be established. Accreditation describes 'the situation wherein the acquisition of certain relevant knowledge, skills and experience enables the practitioner to enhance his/her contribution and either move from one level to another or to qualify for additional reward'. Implicit in this definition is that the registered nurse should have a period of professional consolidation and development following registration and prior to applying for a Staff Nurse post. Most District Health Authorities have since established some form of professional development for their newly registered nurses. All accept the principle of a continuous educational process, many have developed training programmes covering professional consolidation and development in designated training areas but none, so far, have ratified the principle of accreditation. At present, professional development courses in three districts in England are being evaluated by the Department of Health and Social Security and several other districts are observing this exercise closely.

It seems certain that in the not too distant future a new professional structure for nursing will be realized, starting with a core professional module for the newly registered nurse. With the principle of accreditation ratified, successful completion of this module would qualify the nurse to take up a Staff Nurse post, or move on to further post-basic clinical and statutory courses. It is envisaged that each step up the clinical career ladder will be preceded by planned preparation courses with appropriate accreditation.

The professional future of the newly registered nurse depends above all on the individual herself. Nurse managers, through appraisal and performance review can assist in identifying continuing education needs; nurse educators can arrange courses, study days, seminars to meet these needs; but only the nurse herself can use the opportunities provided to improve her knowledge, skills and attitudes ultimately to give high quality care to her patients. Futhermore, even if not wishing to climb the career ladder, the onus is on the individual constantly to appraise and seek appraisal of her performance and progress and to make appropriate moves to meet identified needs. This includes not only attending prescribed courses and study sessions, but also undertaking private reading and joining professional interest groups such as Research and Computers on Nursing. Practising midwives must undertake a refresher course every 5 years and the same is recommended for nurse teachers. It is not inconceivable that some form of continuing education will become mandatory for all nurses and linked to a system of re-registration at stipulated intervals.

What next?

What next then for the newly registered nurse? Just as the budding explorer acquires from the Home Office a passport at the beginning of an exploring career, so the newly qualified nurse acquires from the 'Professional Home Office' – the UKCC – a licence to practise at the beginning of a nursing career. With the passport comes notes for the traveller aimed at producing up-to-date awareness of journeying abroad and safe conduct through foreign lands; with the licence to practise comes guidance for the nurse – a Code of Professional Conduct – aimed at producing up-to-date awareness of professional ethics and safe standards of care. A passport has to be periodically renewed, for a fee; so too with a licence to practise. If the passport is not defaced or defrauded and travelling guidelines are adhered to the explorer will always be eligible for renewal of his passport to travel in safety; if the licence to practise is not defaced or defrauded and the professional code is adhered to, the nurse will always be eligible to re-license in order to travel professionally in safety, giving high quality care.

References

Auld et al. (1981) *Report on Continuing Education for the Nursing Profession in Scotland.* Edinburgh.

Bendall, E. (1975) *So You Passed, Nurse.* RCN Research Series.

Chapman, C. (1977) Concepts of Professionalism. *Journal of Advanced Nursing.* No. 2, pp. 51–55.

Department of Health and Social Security. *Report on Seminar – Professional Development in Clinical Nursing: The 1980s.*

Henderson, V. (1964) The nature of nursing. *American Journal of Nursing* Vol. 64 (No. 8), p. 63.

National Staff Committee for Nurses and Midwives (1981) *The Organisation and Provision of Continuing In-Service Education and Training.*

Pyne, R.H. (1981) *Professional Discipline in Nursing Theory and Practice.* Blackwell Scientific.

Simms, S. (1977) Nursing's Dilemma – the battle for role determination. *Supervisor Nurses* (Sept.), pp. 29–31.

United Kingdom Central Council (1984) *Code of Professional Conduct,* 2nd edn.

Further reading

Department of Health and Social Security. *Where do I go from here?*

Useful addresses

English National Board Post Basic Clinical Nursing Studies Courses: Continuing Education and Training Dept., English National Board for Nursing, Midwifery and Health Visiting, Victory House, 170 Tottenham Court Road, London, W1P 0HA.

English National Board Statutory Post Basic Courses: English National Board for Nursing, Midwifery and Health Visiting, Victory House, 170 Tottenham Court Road, London W1P 0HA

Professional Development and Career Opportunities: Nursing & Health Service Careers Centre, 121/123 Edgware Road, London W2 2HX.

Index

Index

129

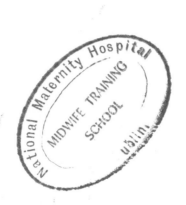